THE ULTIMATE BIRTH EXPERIENCE

How to Take Control and Proactively Choose the Birthing Options That are Best for You and Your Baby

GAIL JANICOLA

First published by Ultimate World Publishing 2021
Copyright © 2021 Gail Janicola

ISBN

Paperback: 978-1-922497-82-6
Ebook: 978-1-922497-83-3

Cover design: Ultimate World Publishing
Layout and typesetting: Ultimate World Publishing
Editor: Isabelle Russell
Cover image: Gus Andi-Shutterstock.com

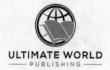

Ultimate World Publishing
Diamond Creek,
Victoria Australia 3089
www.writeabook.com.au

PRAISE

"Planning for, creating, and having an ultimate birth experience does not just happen spontaneously, just as we do not all of a sudden wake up knowledgeable and empowered. It takes active participation and very often, a knowledgeable guide to shepherd our thoughts and our intentions into becoming the experiences that we want for ourselves and our families. I am beyond blessed that Gail has been that guide for my husband and me, helping empower us to have two incredibly beautiful births, as a team and true partners, which led us into parenthood, not just as a mother and a father, but as a family. *The Ultimate Birth Experience* is the roadmap to help you find your guide and embrace the journey as much as the destination."

**Erin Meijer, Moms On Top client,
mother of two amazing kids**

"I was *the* skeptical partner. When my wife told me she didn't want drugs during birth I am pretty sure my reply was, "Well, then can I have them?!" Going through Gail's childbirth education course not only helped me learn so much that I didn't know about pregnancy, labor and delivery but also opened my eyes to why it was so important to my wife. Now I hear her tell the story of our births and she reveres me as the "best labor and delivery husband-coach" she could have ever imagined. I'll take that title all day long and I am so incredibly grateful that we have been on this journey together. I would tell every expecting dad how worth it it is."

DJ Meier, Moms On Top client, Rockstar dad

"Gail is the coach we all wish we had. In this book, she challenges with intellectual dexterity while she nurtures with maternal encouragement. If only more birthing people knew that at the table of decision makers, *they* are at the head. Gail won't let you forget it. If only more birthing people knew that customizing their birth is not too much to ask. Through stories and her own experiences, Gail points out how the pre-canned version of birth often leaves the birthing momma with questions and doubts. She points out how personalization is in fact scientific. Her reverence for science is only matched by her reverence for one's own knowing. She's the wise woman that emboldens you to know your "precious heart and your sacred mind", to get in touch with your needs and become an informed consumer of obstetric services. When a woman listens to her knowing and honors it, she rises from birth a beast of the most exquisite sort – no matter how baby made its debut. This book draws our attention to this transformational power of birth. Sincere, without judgment, Gail cheers you on to own your birth. And if you let her, she'll cheer you on to own your life."

Kathy Shamoun,
Founder, True Birth, Doula, Licensed Acupuncturist

"I've had the privilege of being coached by Gail personally, but for those who are not quite as lucky, this book is the next best thing. Gail has flawlessly combined her wisdom and expertise with genuine compassion, personal experiences, and even some humor. Her loving and caring maternal personality leaps off the pages. You'll see, it's literally impossible not to love her."

Robyn Lanci, Moms On Top student, Doula client

"Knowledge truly is power in birth, as Gail Janicola so beautifully articulates in *The Ultimate Birth Experience*. She argues how important it is to know your options and to advocate for yourself so you can have the birth of your dreams - even if it isn't the birth you planned. I had the pleasure of working with Gail as my birth coach and the lessons she instilled upon me - the very same that you can find here in this book - helped me to handle a birth that was not what I had planned, but that I am at peace with because I was able to make the decisions that were important to me along the way. Bringing a human being into the world is a transformative experience and I urge any woman going through it to take the time to read the *The Ultimate Birth Experience*, as the lessons provided are invaluable and will serve you in birth and beyond."

Chelsea Kocis Trombino, Moms On Top client

Gail has a warm, loving, endless energy to her that wraps you up the moment you are in her presence. And in this book, you feel that energy as she invites you into her world of birth preparation.

The Ultimate Birth Experience goes beyond the typical "natural" birth preparation manual and offers a direct, pull-no-punches analysis and instruction guide to navigating the American maternal healthcare system. Gail urges you to look past the tired divide of women into arbitrary groups according to their birth wishes. She brings us all together as people tuning into our own power and demanding the care we deserve during our births. She goes beyond step-by-step instructions on how to get through labor and slices to the heart of the issues plaguing our failing healthcare system.

Within these pages is a call to action for women everywhere to take control of their births, and get exactly the care they want and deserve for their ultimate birth experience. Not only is this a book that every expecting parent should read, but one that we should share with our obstetricians and midwives as well.

Kaitlin McGreyes, Founder of BeHerVillage.com

For my mom, who loved and supported me unconditionally, and who instilled and nurtured my awe of birth, initiating the greatest ripple effect of my life.

CONTENTS

FOREWORD

I am a woman, wife, mother, grandmother, nurse, childbirth educator and midwife. I have spent more than half my life providing care to women, mothers and infants. I became a midwife to better advocate for women in their healthcare choices, as I became increasingly frustrated with not being able to do so in my role as their nurse. Somewhere along this journey, and many years ago, I met Gail. Gail's incredible passion to raise awareness and provide support to those seeking the kind of care I aspire to provide created an immediate bond. And so, I am incredibly honored and pleased to open the door to *The Ultimate Birth Experience.*

After decades of providing gynecologic and obstetric care, to some who have had positive past experiences but to many who have not, I am convinced that Gail's message of empowerment is an amazing and invaluable gift. She shares insights into many aspects of developing a blueprint for your birth that are supported by science but driven by personal choice. She encourages you to create a community of likeminded support by investing time into the soul searching so critical to revealing your personal birth "tool kit". She persuades you to explore deeply the options available so you can make informed decisions throughout your birth journey while raising awareness that strength, flexibility and acceptance may be needed when the original path is altered by forces beyond your control.

Gail draws on a wealth of knowledge and shares intimate life experiences to successfully motivate your investment in this effort. *The Ultimate Birth Experience* urges you to embrace your instinctive sense of body and self, to trust your innate ability to birth and to expect respect and support of personal choice and protection for the intimacy and sacredness of this magnificent life event.

Dr. Christina Kocis CNM, FACNM
Director – Midwifery Division, Department of Obstetrics and Gynecology
Stony Brook University Hospital
Stony Brook, New York

INTRODUCTION

Think of all the times you have moved through an experience and found yourself changed on the other side; times where you looked back in hindsight and realized how your thoughts and beliefs shifted in a way you could not have imagined. Every valuable moment of growth in your life depends on your experiences. The experience of birth is especially powerful, but that power is often unrecognized until it's too late; until that moment of hindsight mocks you for not paying attention.

Whether you are in the contemplation stage of starting a family, at the precipice of having your first baby, or preparing to give birth again, you deserve the massive rewards that begin with an open mind and the desire to take control and become empowered. If you take action in designing your ultimate birth experience using the guidance in this book, you will very likely avoid needing resources to work through a *traumatic* birth experience in the future.

My goal is to help you reconnect your mind to your body and to embrace the fact that childbirth is a part of the flow of life. I hope you will question and analyze and take as much responsibility as possible. My intention is for you to feel stronger after giving birth than you ever have before.

The objective is to enlighten you, not to sway you or convince you to feel something you do not feel about birth. It is most certainly to give you the means by which to actualize whatever it is that is important to you. YOU - not me, not your best friend, or your mother, or anyone else.

You may already know much of what I uncover, or you may be blown away by some of the concepts and truths I share. Either way, you will arrive at a place where you have clarity around your beliefs, thoughts, wants and needs, and where you are motivated to take action.

The ultimate birth experience is one in which _____ . You get to fill in the blank. But not yet. Not until you have the tools to explore everything from your own values to our cultural history, from your personal points of view to the most credible evidence. Once you do this, you may end up in the same exact place you are right now, with the same exact perspectives, but I doubt it.

It is probable that your vantage point is about to shift to some degree – like being on the runway in an airplane where you can only see what is right outside your window, and then taking off and visualizing details like grids of houses, patches of water, and tracks of roadways spanning long distances and circling in intricate connections. When you're on the ground you cannot see any of this, but once you reach a higher elevation, your view is more expansive. That's my purpose – to give you the ability to reach that higher elevation, to see wide and clear; the platform on which you can take control, make the safest, best choices, and become empowered now and forevermore. Your sense of self, what you know about birth, the decisions you make in preparation and during the process, and how you are treated throughout, can be life-changing.

Chapter 1

NO ONE WAY

"However much we know about birth in general, we know nothing about a particular birth. We must let it unfold with its own uniqueness."

— ELIZABETH NOBLE

We are advanced, as both a species and a culture. We *know* so much, and we *have* so much. If someone had told us, just 20 years ago, that someday we would be able to type an address – any address in the entire world - into our handheld computers (which would also be our phones, music players, and better cameras than the ones professional photographers were currently using) and they would, within seconds, map out our rides with not only written directions, but with 3-dimensional graphics, including icons for gas stations, restaurants, and hidden police cars, we might not have believed them.

Science and technology progress constantly. Nothing stays the same for very long, and because of that we can barely remember "what it used to be like". With current ways replacing old ways at lightning speed, often furnishing us with conveniences we never thought possible, we become mesmerized, infatuated and addicted to the new and improved, in a way that doesn't allow us to believe that anything but the latest and greatest could be worthwhile.

Because of this, we discount alternatives. We ignore the possibility that there could be more than one way, maybe even a better way. We see in black and white. This way good, that way bad. After all, look how far we've come! Why would anyone want to go backwards? If the technology exists, it must be making our lives the best they could be, and we must be the safest we've ever been. Therefore, doing it any other way, choosing any other options, would be crazy. And we're just not going to tolerate that!

We have taken the most personal experience in our lives and homogenized it with blind faith on the assumption that high-tech progress is synonymous with the ideal, the best, the safest.

Sadly, this is precisely the mindset around birth. We have taken the most personal experience in our lives and homogenized it with blind faith on the assumption that high-tech progress is synonymous with the ideal, the best, the safest.

And so, dear unique being, you may have been convinced that there is only one way to have a baby, and that this one way includes rules and protocols, checklists, and schedules. You might not have even considered that there was a way that might be better for you because that would be blasphemy – to question the advancements that, in theory, could keep you and your baby safe from harm.

What if I told you that it's not that clear cut? That there are so many more aspects and angles that you are possibly unaware of? Positions that would give you the space to explore a variety of options until you came up with what you wanted and felt was right and best for you?

We will talk more about the truth behind the science, but let's start with some common sense around simple physiology. Your body is different than anyone else's body on the entire planet, pregnant or otherwise. Yes, your anatomy during pregnancy has some special features that are shared by all others who are pregnant, but there are, still, many distinctions - just as there can be controllable differences in your biology. Investing in your health and wellness with sound lifestyle choices sets you apart from those who choose to believe that eating double the calories, passing on daily exercise, and burning the candle at both ends, are appropriate behaviors during pregnancy. You may have some pre-existing conditions, or experience certain developments that would put you in a high-risk category, but the way you treat your body can have an influence on how those conditions and developments play out in pregnancy and birth.

Certainly, when it comes to labor and birth experiences, no two will ever be alike, whether you're comparing yours to someone else's or making the comparison between two of your own. It is just not possible for birth to unfold the same exact way every time, for every person. And so, you should expect your care to

9

be individualized instead of thinking that it is suitable to fit your birth into a predetermined blueprint.

Putting aside the physical and the science for a moment more, I ask you this: what about the experience of giving birth is important to you? You're not allowed to answer with "having a healthy baby". That goes without saying. Try to go deeper. This may be a challenging question, considering that there is, generally, very little regard for one's values, desires, and perspectives when it comes to birth. You might not have ever examined this side of the equation, but I'm here to tell you, right now, that this is the greatest missing link to the ultimate birth experience. This suppression, and sometimes flat-out disdain for the psychological, social, emotional, and spiritual sides of what constitutes a good birth, is one reason why people are either dissatisfied with their births or have a sort of apathetic stance. Without tapping into your intimate principles when reflecting on this journey of a lifetime, you will never discover that you have options, you will not be supported as an individual, you won't know how to, and more importantly, *why* you need to plan your birth – and you will miss out on every lifelong opportunity this experience will create. This is the foundation. Seeing yourself as a singular soul is the catalyst for perceiving the concept of "no one way" in birth.

If you could not come up with an answer to the question of what is important to you, other than "having a healthy baby", I fully respect that. Not every person cares to be submerged in deep thinking around birth. You may be quite content with going no further than securing a safe birth. If that is you, read on. I believe you will begin to grasp the association between developing underlying beliefs and specific wants around birth, and reducing risks; between discovering what you, indirectly, care about, and improving the outcome for your baby, and for you. Just maybe, at that point, you'll begin to see some other benefits to individualizing your birth experience, but no pressure, and certainly no judgment if not.

Science upholds the idea of differentiating birth practices because science knows we are each physiologically different to some extent, and it has revealed the benefits and the risks of medical interventions. The basic conclusion has always been that the cons will outweigh the pros and the potential risks will outweigh potential benefits when any protocol, procedure or intervention is administered to someone who is pregnant or during labor in a *routine* fashion. For instance, if you are having a normal, low-risk labor, there is no medical need for the routine protocol of having you lie in bed. So, then, the potential benefits of being out of bed, including facilitating the progress of labor with gravity and the shifting of your pelvis, would outweigh the nonexistent risks. Conversely, if your blood pressure dropped significantly, and you were feeling dizzy, the benefits of upright positions and movement would still exist, but they would not eclipse the risks. No longer would lying in bed be a routine practice, but one that was medically necessary. Do you see the distinction and how you might use this to decide what was best for you if your goal was a safe birth, one that progressed easily, without complications?

Every pregnant person is going to have a unique labor experience. Some may be similar but no two will be exactly the same. Using a checklist of routine interventions to manage a labor is like wearing a winter coat on a summer day just in case the temperature drops suddenly. It's not a bad idea to bring a sweater if you're going to a chilly supermarket or an air-conditioned restaurant, but until you get there, you don't know if you'll actually need it, and in the meantime, you're overheating because you have on a down jacket and it's 80 degrees!

Please always be authentically yourself, especially when considering your birth experience. Your journey through birth is as unique as your journey through life. Each person's circumstances are different. Feeling acknowledged and having your hopes and dreams and expectations heard, respected, and validated will promote an empowered birth experience. Receiving personalized care, where your needs and preferences are valued, will provide you with a strong sense of dignity and control during a particularly vulnerable time. To achieve your goals, as extensive or minimal as they may be, support is crucial. The understanding by those who will support you in labor, that you are an individual, having a very personal, individualized birth, will increase the level, the sincerity, and the significance of that support, and subsequently raise the likelihood of realizing the birth you hope to have. The power of making decisions that suit you best – knowing that *you* are the only one who can make those decisions for yourself and your baby – where you're connecting those decisions to your own values, defines living your truth. This is the way to foster confidence in your birth experience, and as a jumping-off point for the rest of your life.

Don't lump yourself in the same category as everyone else. When you ignore or deny what is most meaningful for you in order to be a good daughter, student, friend, or patient, you end up missing the cues that mobilize mental, physical, and emotional health and well-being. You give up control. You give up your rights to your own body, and to your own baby. You essentially tell others that they know what is best for you, and, as a result, you may end up with outcomes you never expected – standard outcomes that evolved from standard practices, meant for satisfying the expectations of others. As the great Jim Rohn (entrepreneur, author, and motivational speaker) once said: "If you don't design your own life plan, chances are you'll fall into someone else's plan. And guess what they have planned for you? Not much." It's not that this "someone else" doesn't care. This is not about bashing your sister, your mother-in-law, or your doctor. Their kindness and love for you could be extraordinary, but they are not you. Their ideas and beliefs, behaviors and actions are for each of them, for the realization of *their* goals, not yours.

Although I was birth-ignorant during my first two pregnancies, and, consequently, could not make many of the choices that would secure all that was important to me, I knew I was in love with the idea of being pregnant and giving birth. I cared deeply about the experience, but I left all the crucial components of my wish list to chance, assuming there was only one way. I did no research and took a class that prepared me for protocols – checklists that were created for the benefit and agendas of others; systems put in place for an administrative process. I never considered the idea that every person giving birth was truly unique and required a deeper understanding and acknowledgment of both the natural evolution of this grand physiological event, and preparation for the various choices they would be faced with in the moment. I wanted to fit in. I didn't want to make waves. I assumed things would go "well", which they did, because I was lucky. I assumed I would be joyful, which I was, because it's who I am. My level of comfort relied solely on my doctor's personality and her credentials. In later years, my husband and I would marvel at how it would take us weeks to buy a blender because we needed to first pore over Consumer Reports, but we accepted every aspect of birth at face value, barely asking questions outside of whether we should park in the garage or pull up to the emergency room. We knew that the birth of our baby was infinitely more important than which blenders had the best features, but we shrugged off our researching responsibility in favor of allowing the experts to assume authority. What we failed to recognize was that *we* were the experts.

SEE YOURSELF AS A CONSUMER WITH CHOICES

Would you ever get engaged, hire a wedding planner and let them choose every aspect of your wedding – every detail of *your* wedding day?

Imagine if you were buying a home and were not given the choice of what kind of structure you could purchase. There was just one size, one neighborhood. No distinctions like two-floor colonial versus one-level ranch, or apartment versus mansion. No choices between rural or urban, tree-lined with backyards, or skyscrapers with rooftops. No options such as central A/C, gas cooktops, and garages or parking spaces. As a consumer, would you accept a standard protocol for your home, especially if your intention was to plant roots for years to come?

The broader issue here is that we not only ignore our roles as the experts in our births, when we would most definitely consider ourselves experts in other areas of our lives, fully aware of our needs, but we also neglect to see ourselves as *consumers* in our births, the way we most definitely see ourselves in most other situations. If you take a moment to define what being a consumer means to you, I think you'd include certain expectations, like being given the opportunity to gather your own information and anticipate receiving further information from the skilled associates you choose for your transaction. You would probably not be comfortable with vital knowledge that would influence your decision-making being withheld from you, and I'm figuring you would walk away from any interaction in which you were being pressured or coerced or misled. And how about those choices? I'm going to bet that you would look at a realtor like they had three heads if they said, "no need for discussions about what you want. No, I don't need to see your wish list. That's not how I do things. At Realty XYZ we offer one type of dwelling only. We like it best. It works for us. Most people have no problem with it. Don't be difficult."

Wowza. That would suck, and you would not stand for it, because it makes no sense, it's ridiculous, and it's insulting. Oh, and by the way, now that you are embarking on this other experience, where you will bring forth life and transform yourself forever - which might just be a little (or a *lot*) more high-stakes than buying a home, the role you need to see yourself in is that of... you guessed it ... a consumer. Do not be okay with having information concealed and being told that your wish list is a waste of time. Do not accept pressure, coercion, and deception. And, certainly, do not consent to the idea that you are just like everyone else and there is only one way.

Specific to birth, this goes in two directions. I am not only talking to those who aim to have natural births, with no medication or interventions. Because items like epidurals and inductions are typically part of

What matters is that your choices, based on your values and, preferably, made with the knowledge of evidence-based information, are supported and honored, and separated from hidden agendas and judgment.

the standard list, as opposed to the individualized list, the need to advocate for what you want usually applies more to those who would prefer to avoid those things. But, in the end, that doesn't matter. What matters is that your choices, based on your values and, preferably, made with the knowledge of evidence-based information, are supported and honored, and separated from hidden agendas and judgment.

KNOWLEDGE IS INDEED POWER

If you're still shrugging your shoulders, in part because the idea of sorting through your beliefs and wishes around birth seems too abstract for you, I would suggest starting with the education piece first. It often happens that when you accumulate knowledge and become more enlightened, epiphanies occur, causing you to gain new thoughts around what you are learning and immersing yourself in. What is that you say? You are too busy working and getting ready for this baby that you don't have the time, not to mention the funds, to take classes? Rest assured, you are in good company, and I'm certainly not going to be the one to preach to you and add more stress to your already stressful life. But since I know the education part can be a game changer, and because you found me and you're trusting me enough to lean in here, I'll gently suggest that you figure this part out. Find resources you can listen to while walking, exercising, driving, or otherwise commuting to and from work. I would caution against going down the Google rabbit hole. As convenient and cost effective as it might be, I advise against this. You're wise enough to know that not everything you find on a search engine is researched and evidence-based, much less accurate and unbiased, so it goes without saying that you should, at least, seek out information that is. Basic, irrefutable facts aside, like your anatomy during pregnancy, it's not that easy to find comprehensive, fact-based birth information, over opinions and prejudice. It's also not that easy to find articles that will encourage you to see different sides and make this your own, which will just leave you where you were before – without the ability to tap into your personal mindset around birth, and individualize your thoughts, beliefs, and wishes. Occasionally, with time spent doing extensive searching, you can qualify authors, bloggers, journalists, and their sources, and it's possible to pull up some reputable pieces. However, you don't exactly have time for that. That's part of the issue. I'm presuming you don't exactly have the inclination either. So, my gold-standard suggestion would be to find someone who believes in the "no one way" philosophy. Someone you relate to and feel you can place your confidence in, who will provide some flexibility on the time and money issues and can impart the learning and coaching that will set you on the path to an empowered and potentially life-changing birth experience. Yup, it's just that valuable.

Be critical of which books you choose to read as well. No slight on the publication itself, but I have a visceral reaction to the phrase "what to *expect* when you're expecting", as this implies that there is one, standard way, universally experienced by all pregnant people, to traverse through the very diverse journey of creating a human. As if you can and *should* know in advance what your particular path will look like. It removes the possibility of individualizing your experience, overlooking the fact that pregnancy is the time in your life when you will physically and mentally be the *most* distinguished. This "what to expect" concept is flawed as it relates to birth as well, for it seals the deal on the erroneous, empowerment-sucking idea that there is a standard, best way to give birth to a baby, emphasizing your lack of choice.

Yes, there are general developments and happenings that unfold during most pregnancies. I concede that it can be helpful to know what you *might* be experiencing, and fun to know which fruit your baby's size correlates to at various milestones throughout your pregnancy. Honestly, I'm not trying to be a buzzkill! However, the idea of "what to expect" is deceiving, and it further perpetuates this notion that all expecting people feel the same, look the same, want the same, and will have the same experience. It doesn't address the nuances, and it doesn't suggest the existence of options and rights.

COMMUNICATE WITH STRENGTH AND DIPLOMACY

I've had these discussions with many people over many years, and I've been able to impress on them the importance of it all, to influence their commitment and self- assurance, only to have it unraveled by well-meaning family and friends, or shattered by fear and intimidation at the thought of approaching their doctors and other medical providers.

If you are feeling pressured by someone in your life who just loves you and only wants the best for you, or maybe a family member or friend who simply feels compelled to brow beat you with their opinions about birth and possibly their entire worldview, try to take a step back, observe with curiosity, don't get defensive, and hear them out. And then, move on. What a wonderful opportunity to sharpen the skill of maintaining boundaries. If, instead of getting flustered and upset, you spend a few seconds understanding where they might be coming from – whether it's a place of love or concern, or a personal unmet need to be "right" – you are gifting them with being heard *and* you're also standing firm in the trust you have in yourself. Communicate how much you appreciate them, only entering into a full discussion if they are open to that, and not just being a filibuster, ignoring or rejecting what you have to say. Either way, continue to march in your own parade.

As far as doctors and other medical providers are concerned, try the same approach. Before shrinking at the very thought of a discussion about your birth, seek to understand where their concerns and beliefs come from. Again, observe with curiosity. Ego and possible hidden agendas aside, their goal is a healthy outcome for you and your baby. The lack of understanding around the influence that individualizing birth has on that outcome might be what is missing from the equation.

Remember this: the "how" of communication is equally as important as the "what". If you either bow to the altar of the MD, or, conversely, you enter the conversation with guns blazing, you will not have a productive or pleasant outcome. So, consider this one piece of advice. First, muster up and display confidence, recognizing that you absolutely know what's best for you, especially with science on your side. You don't have to know medical lingo in order to communicate intelligently, and you don't have to impress your doctor in order to justify your truth. Second, convey your thoughts, your preferences, and your needs with a calm demeanor. And third, ask for support in realizing your goals and dreams. It is unlikely that you will be met with defensiveness and scorn if you simply request the human decency of respect for your individual choices, especially if you include your intention to be flexible in

You don't have to know medical lingo in order to communicate intelligently, and you don't have to impress your doctor in order to justify your truth.

unpredictable circumstances. The way in which you conduct yourself will lead and set the tone for the conversation. If your individuality is still devalued, you can remind yourself that you, as a consumer of healthcare, are always in the driver's seat.

An extremely important thought to hold onto is that you will cling to the memory of this birth in your heart and mind for the rest of your life. You will re-live every detail. It will change you – hopefully, in the most profoundly positive of ways. However, no one else, except maybe your partner, will hold the memory of this birth in *their* hearts and minds for the rest of *their* lives. Your doctor or midwife, doula and nurses may be a huge part of your experience as you journey through the months of pregnancy and hours of labor, but they will absolutely forget the details of your story and the vast majority of stories they are a part of. Imagine then, the tragic insignificance of giving in and giving up your priceless autonomy so as not to ruffle feathers or make waves.

Stand strong and speak up. Share what is in your precious heart and sacred mind. It will be the most beautiful and meaningful song you ever sing, and you'll begin to sing it over and over again. Despite the unease you may experience during confrontation, I guarantee you will not die if you have an unpleasant encounter - one that actually turns out to be truly intimidating - even after you prepared and put your plan into action. You will learn from this. You will grow from this. You will become stronger, and you will likely become the most enthusiastic defender of individuality in birth. You will also be even more convinced that there is no one way to have a baby.

WHAT NOW?

○ Spend time pondering what the meaning of the ultimate birth experience is to you. Understand that birth is important for each person in a different way.

○ Expect your feelings to be validated at all times, even when there are opposing points of view.

○ Surround yourself with those who understand the immense importance of "no one way" when it comes to birth, and distance yourself from those who don't.

○ Read books and follow websites and blogs that provide evidence-based information and normalize birth.

○ Learn from studies on the Evidence Based Birth® website. (https://evidencebasedbirth.com/)

○ Practice communicating calmly and confidently. Pay attention to your tone (firm and unapologetic) and always show appreciation. When you eventually have conversations with your family, friends and medical providers, you will feel more comfortable asking for what you want and less likely to accept "what she's having" so as not to make waves.

Thoughts and Actions

_____

_____

_____

_____

_____

_____

_____

_____

_____

_____

_____

_____

_____

Chapter 2

THE RISK OF IGNORANCE

"If you don't know your options, you don't have any."
– DIANA KORTE & ROBERTA SCAER

For over 25 years I have been told "if I had only known you when I was pregnant" more times than I can remember. This disclosure usually comes after any situation in which I find myself talking about pregnancy and birth, whether I'm being asked what I do, or at times when I'm part of a group of women who are mothers - anywhere, anytime, at any age - as this topic has a way of sneaking itself into some of the most unrelated exchanges.

Although seemingly complimentary, I come away feeling deeply frustrated. I believe things happen the way they're supposed to, in the time they're supposed to, and yet, the thought that someone's birth experience could have been improved in any way; the idea that an interaction with me, or exposure to information could have prevented a birth trauma, is unfortunate and discouraging all the same. If I've said it once, to my students and others, I've said it a million times: "Don't have regret. Do everything in your power to live a regret-free life." As the serenity prayer says, "God, grant me the strength to accept the things I cannot change, courage to change the things I can, and wisdom to know the difference". Sadly, it's public opinion that one cannot change *anything* in birth. Mustering the strength needed for acceptance is not all that difficult, and courage doesn't seem necessary when you feel you have no command over how things play out. When you're led to believe you have no control, acceptance and courage are meaningless. Wisdom never enters the picture at all, and serenity is then pretty elusive. What you're likely to be left with is regret. That's the risk of ignorance.

THERE'S NO SHAME IN IGNORANCE

I created the 'Birth IQ quiz', a collection of 12 multiple-choice questions, to assess someone's knowledge of birth. (To take the quiz, refer to page 201.) The objective behind its conception was not to determine whether or not you know inconsequential facts of birth, but whether or not you could apply accurate facts to master your birth experience. For example, your ability to choose the correct answer to, "If the baby is having trouble descending into the pelvis during the first stage of labor, you should"... indicates that you understand the following:

1. How your pelvis works during labor; and
2. Your influence over how your pelvis works during labor.

Knowing this answer would, in very real and common situations that arise during birth, give you the ability to make choices that could affect the outcome of your labor.

The point of the quiz is to either prove that you already have the knowledge to distinguish between myths and facts, and control what you can during the birth process, or that you don't. If you don't, that's ok - at least for now. I do want you to recognize how detrimental it would be to stay ignorant as you walk into your birth, and how empowering it would be to be able to acquire the knowledge that could make a huge difference in your experience, but I certainly understand that it can be overwhelming when it comes to where to begin on the path to learning, understanding and preparing. Think of this simple quiz as your roadmap on the journey toward gaining more and more knowledge.

After hundreds of people had taken this quiz, I received some unexpected feedback. Many low scorers were insulted. Instead of thinking "wow, there was so much I didn't know going into my labor that could have influenced what happened", or "wow, I need to get this information before I go into labor", I received defensive comments like "this quiz is B.S., I have five children so I think I know how to give birth", and "who cares if my score is low? You don't have any control over what happens anyway." I was shocked. These reactions confirmed that our maternity culture has really done a number on us. For people to be so certain that they still have no agency over their own bodies and their own experiences, even *after* showing them that they do, and that people will close their minds with a padlock in order to protect their egos, is baffling.

Just as the mistakes you make and the failures you experience can help you to learn, to grow, to get better, and do better, ignorance can work in a similar way. Ignorance is more subtle than failure though. Failure is obvious, but ignorance takes an enlightened awareness. You have to realize that you don't know what you don't know, and then, of course, you have to see the value in reversing that. There is no shame in being ignorant, at least not if you attempt not to be. Ignorance does not mean "stupid". All it means is that you don't know something *yet*. As a general rule of thumb, what we don't know far outweighs what we do know. Pursuing knowledge is a great practice – one I passionately endorse, and one I'll spend plenty of time discussing with you. There will always be so much you don't know for many reasons, one of which might be lack of need. If you don't have a need to know about something, then, by all means, don't waste your time studying it. But, even if you have no intention of integrating a specific topic into your life's work, it would still be worthwhile to gain some knowledge if it could personally be of benefit to you at a particular juncture along your path. You don't have to aspire to be an automobile mechanic, but if you want to drive a car it would be a good idea to know how to work a gas pump. In the same way, you do not have to return to school to earn credentials as a midwife or obstetrician in order to gain an advantage from some degree of knowledge about pregnancy and birth if you happen to be pregnant and you're going to give birth.

Remaining ignorant, when it's a choice on your part – one that doesn't cause a fallout or a roadblock to your well-being – seems fair. That is not the case when it comes to birth - anyone's birth, regardless of medical status (low-risk or high-risk). When all those women expressed misgiving at not, somehow, making my acquaintance when they were pregnant, what they were really suggesting was disappointment in "not knowing" period, for it's not me, but the information received comprehensively, without judgment, that grants the opportunity for a better, safer, more empowered birth experience. I am not a fairy godmother, magically making this happen for birthing women. The power lies within to seek and find the resources that educate, inform, uplift, and strengthen.

THE WORTH OF CHILDBIRTH EDUCATION AND WHY IT'S UNDERVALUED

Childbirth education can be exceptionally valuable, yet the idea of childbirth education has been watered-down, stereotyped and parodied. It began with good intentions in 1960, with The Lamaze® method emerging after Margie Karmel gave birth, assisted by Dr. Fernand Lamaze, and she wrote of her experience in the book *Thank You Dr. Lamaze*. This time in history was ripe for change in birthing practices, as women latched onto the feminist movement in the 60s subculture. Childbirth classes were a way to receive information that was essentially hidden from pregnant women who needed it the most. Within this process of taking control was a very strong statement of equality, of power over one's own body, and rights in childbirth. Change did take place. As is the case in almost every large-scale evolution, a sweeping, organized effort was the spark that started the engine, and, ultimately, ignited the fuel that gave it power. This organized effort made changes to both the mindset of women during pregnancy and the maternity system as a whole. Partners were now invited into delivery rooms and renewed support for breastfeeding was developing.

The response to this initiation has grown in functional ways, with progression taking place within the physical structure of hospitals. No longer do women give birth in sterile operating rooms. They

THE ULTIMATE BIRTH EXPERIENCE

labor, give birth, and recover all in the same space. This change has occurred in the time since I began my career, during the time I was having my babies – a relatively recent 20-25 years ago. With the force behind the women's movement, businesses such as hospitals were pressured into making these changes; alterations that have continued steadily. Unfortunately, this revolution did not follow an upward trajectory in all aspects. We experienced a constructive swing of the pendulum, but even with the continued beautifying of labor rooms and the acceptance of doulas in those rooms as professional sources of support, the advancements in technology have exerted a vigorous pull on women and our birth culture as a whole. Momentum has ceased, and in many ways, we have slipped backwards.

Instead of childbirth classes serving to educate and empower, they became entrenched in the hospital system as efficient platforms for preparing expectant parents for hospital protocols and routines. With the surge in reliance on technology, this is what women signed up for and in fact preferred. They weren't looking to reduce their anxiety around birth by actually learning how to manage labor, because they were seduced by the promise of having their labor managed for them. They just wanted to know what entrance to navigate when they arrived at the hospital, and how soon they could get an epidural. This dichotomy between the original purpose of childbirth education and what largely exists today is incredibly sad.

Instead of childbirth classes serving to educate and empower, they became entrenched in the hospital system as efficient platforms for preparing expectant parents for hospital protocols and routines.

Women have been stripped of the power they had longed and fought for. In its place, our culture has created a feeling of omnipotence around medicine, encouraging a sense of reliance and entitlement around birthing women. The common dialogue is as follows:

Birthing person: "Please help me and furnish me with all the high-tech procedures that will make me more comfortable and guarantee safety for me and my baby."

Hospital/Care Provider: "We'll take care of everything."

Basically, we've opened the window and thrown out evidence, options, partnership, independence, personalization, wisdom and advocacy. Some people may say they're okay with this, and if all goes well, they're happy to move on and never look back. But if you want more from the experiences in your life – in this case, your birth - the experience that houses and promotes massive opportunities for lifelong well-being, then you must overcome a sense of complacency or discard distorted beliefs around control and the lack thereof.

MY MOTHER'S STORY – THE BIRTH OF MY BROTHER

When my mother was pregnant, she knew virtually nothing about how her body was working to nurture a growing fetus, or would work during the birth process, or even how to determine whether or not she was in labor. I mean no disrespect to my mother. She was a very intelligent, sophisticated woman, who, in my humble opinion, was an extraordinary mother. She just wasn't educated about pregnancy and birth, for the very same reasons why the majority of modern American women continue to be uneducated about pregnancy and birth.

On a chilly day in October, after fighting an acute illness for a couple of days, my mother started feeling pains in her belly. My grandparents, always concerned about their daughter, who, as a teenager, had suffered heart damage in her mitral valve after a bout of rheumatic fever, came to stay with my parents, and to care for my mom. No one predicted she was in labor, quite possibly, in part because she was four weeks away from her estimated due date. As the morning wore on, the pains became more intense and frequent. She called her obstetrician. He was unavailable for a house call (standard practice in those days) so he sent another doctor - an orthopedist. I'm not certain if Dr. Ortho actually examined her or not. I do know that he checked her medical records and discussed the symptoms of her supposed illness. He then concluded that she was not in labor, but that the "flu had settled in her stomach". And he left. Hours later, when the pains were becoming worse, the OB was called again. Apparently, he was at a dinner party, and asked my dad to bring my mom to meet him at his office. Upon arrival, as he examined her in his tuxedo, he immediately determined that she was in labor. I can't tell you how far along she was or if things were moving quickly, but it was clear that this labor was indeed progressing. During his brief examination, he decided to rupture her membranes (break the amniotic sac of water) and instructed my dad to bring her to the hospital, where he would meet them. It was cold. It was raining. She was soaking wet and running a fever.

Shortly after she arrived at the hospital, my mom became very ill and lost consciousness. It's possible that her somewhat compromised heart function increased the risk of complications.

At one point, there was a brief conversation where the doctor informed my father that there was a chance his wife and his baby might not both survive, and he could, potentially, be called on to make a choice. My poor, distraught dad waited in a room set aside for family members who were expecting happy news, disconnected from the experience as all fathers were in those days, and, I imagine, much more frightened than the others.

No one will ever know the details of what occurred in that delivery room in Brooklyn Jewish Hospital, on the evening of October 20, 1957. I have no doubt that everything possible was done to save both mother and baby; that the highest levels of technology that existed in 1957, and the highest levels of medical knowledge and expertise possessed by my mother's doctor and nurses were implemented. To a certain degree, that is why my mother went on to live a long life that, eventually, included another less dramatic, more typical and joyful birth story. My brother also continues to enjoy a full, although challenging life, because of the efforts in that delivery room.

Until he was four years old, there was never a diagnosis for my brother's failure to thrive. He was delayed in all of the milestones, but typical in appearance, so his pediatrician determined that my mom and dad had "first-time-parent-anxiety" and told them not to worry. Of course they worried. They didn't have medical degrees, but they did have plenty of intelligence and intuition. Eventually, he was deemed to be "brain-injured", and my parents spent the rest of their days doing everything to give him the best life possible.

I can construct endless scenarios for how things could have been different. What if an obstetrician, instead of an orthopedist, came to the apartment? What if my mother had just gone to the hospital and submitted to every intervention possible? What if they had performed a C-section? What if she had just basically lived in the hospital her entire pregnancy? Wasn't it true back then, as it still is today, that *more* is better when it comes to birth?

When I planned to start my own family, I was going to accept, and even request access to every last modern obstetric advancement that existed. I was excited about being pregnant and giving birth and looked forward to the process in its entirety, but I also owned my mother's experience and clung tightly to my assumptions. I believed that the only way to ensure safety was with machines and procedures. I never gave a second thought to advocating for myself or even investigating my options. Living with a disabled brother and internalizing the scenario that led up to his impairment was enough to keep my mind closed to the idea of a so-called "natural" birth, especially if my doctor felt that routine procedures equated with safety.

Less was not more in my mind. More was more and more was better. End of story. That is, until, after two pregnancies and births, when I decided to become a doula and a childbirth educator. Remarkably, upon simply reading as part of my coursework, I began having one "aha" moment after another. It was like there were layers of erroneous beliefs shrouding my story about birth and, bit by bit, I was uncovering revelations that prompted me to ask new questions – questions like, "What if my *mother* had read some of these books?"; "What if she understood her body and the process of labor?"; "What if she recognized that she was in labor, or even questioned whether or not she was, instead of robotically putting her trust in someone else's assessment?"

My mother did the best she could in the moment. I see her, in part, as a victim of her generation and the culture in which we still live; a victim of the lack of value placed on childbirth education and self-advocacy, and the unhealthy burden we, to this day, place on physicians to take care of us. Quite possibly, things would have turned out the same. Who really knows? It's miserable and pointless to play the "what if" game throughout life. Controlling what can be controlled is where the value lies. It does not necessarily offer guarantees, but it affects our ability to live a regret-free life. You can probably further understand now just why that is so important to me, and why I emphasize this with you.

The path to my life as a birth professional opened my mind, provided me with what felt like secret knowledge, and gave me a new perspective. Eventually seeing my brother's birth story in a different light offered an interpretation with much more clarity, and a conviction that influenced my third birth and every part of my life since. To be enamored by the medical school your doctor attended, and the number of medical devices acquired by your hospital, is to be distracted from the vital role you play in your own birth, and to be afflicted with a false sense of security.

> *To be enamored by the medical school your doctor attended, and the number of medical devices acquired by your hospital, is to be distracted from the vital role you play in your own birth, and to be afflicted with a false sense of security.*

What you do to ensure safety and avert a crisis matters first and foremost, for those actions would often intercept the need to be "saved". Just as I am not shaming my mother by believing it was

33

her responsibility to be informed, to understand her body, to trust her instincts, and to take a partnership role in her pregnancy and birth, I am not shaming you when I say it is your responsibility to yourself to do the same. But it is, and you should, if you feel it's important to know the things that could, conceivably, change the trajectory of your birth experience.

TAKING PAGES OUT OF HISTORY

Although time lags or delays in research are estimates, and not well understood, it is frequently stated that it takes an average of 17 years from the time evidence is published until the time it reaches clinical practice.(1) What that means for us is that certain routine medical practices and recommendations we currently take for granted as being safe and effective – drugs and procedures in particular - might have been proven to be unsafe and ineffective years ago, but are still marketed, prescribed, and part of the standard of care. We've seen this numerous times within the specific historical boundaries of pregnancy and birth, which is why the dangerous practice of burying one's head in the sand instead of searching for as much information as possible is confounding.

DES
From about 1940 to 1971, the drug DES was prescribed as a medication to pregnant women who had had previous miscarriages. As it was believed that the cause of some miscarriages was an insufficient level of estrogen, and because DES was a type of estrogen, its purpose was to reduce the risk of pregnancy complications and losses.(2) A study published in 1971 (indicating that the research had to have been done prior to that year) showed

that DES caused a rare type of vaginal cancer in girls and young women who had been exposed to DES when their mothers were pregnant with them. Furthermore, less incriminating research showing that DES did *not* prevent miscarriages or premature births was first published in 1953, 18 years *before* the FDA eventually issued a Drug Bulletin advising physicians to stop prescribing it to pregnant women.(3)

Thalidomide
Although the US averted a major medical disaster with the drug Thalidomide, the effects were devastating (over 10,000 severe birth defects) to babies born in 46 countries around the world, in the late 1950s. It was a sedative that was touted for its ability to relieve morning sickness, marketed heavily and advertised as completely safe until later being banned in 1961. Sample packets were freely distributed to patients.(4)

Smoking
Other seemingly benign recommendations included smoking cigarettes as a way to curb weight gain and manage anxiety during pregnancy. Even when it wasn't necessarily recommended, it was felt to be a safe practice, with the suggested, arbitrary limit of 4 a day. Evidence on the link between lung cancer, heart disease and smoking cigarettes, in general, was presented at the American Medical Association's annual conference in 1954. The results of further studies were the same and led to the Surgeon General's Report on Smoking and Health in 1964.(5) In 1965 warning labels were put on cigarette packaging, 11 years *after* the conclusions that came from the first of the largest prospective studies.

X-Rays

Although every woman, from the time she's an adolescent until well into middle-age, is asked if she could be pregnant before receiving even a small dose of radiation from a dental X-ray, and then given a heavy lead apron to cover her body to shield her from most of that radiation, there was a time when pregnant women were receiving abdominal X-rays as part of routine prenatal screenings. Starting in the 1920s, X-rays were used on pregnant women to determine the size of the pelvis and the size and positioning of the fetus. A high-level study presented evidence of the connection between X-rays and childhood leukemia in 1956. This research was discredited, but later confirmed, along with other studies that showed increases in abnormalities in babies who were exposed to X-rays in utero. X-rays during pregnancy continued into the mid-70s, 20 years *after* that first study.(6)

In conveying these cases, some may argue that we can only follow the medical advice of our time; the medical advice that is known and familiar. To me, that is a cop-out and a defense of the ignorance fan club. I once had an offended student drop my class because they didn't like that I used the example of ultrasound to inspire them to think outside the box. In wanting to invigorate their decision-making muscles, I suggested taking into consideration what we know as facts about the immediate effects of high frequency sound waves on fetuses, when being faced with the persuasion to submit to lots of routine scans – being clear that there is no definitive evidence showing long-term, negative outcomes. The idea was to get them to think before acting, to consider all the facts and potential risks in relation to the benefits, to learn from history and do what so many wish they might have done decades ago, at the time when they were blindly accepting claims of absolute safety around recommendations and routines that we now look back on with shock and disgust.

Either the research is there, and the information does actually exist but it's not known because some hidden agenda is keeping it from you (and me, and the rest of the general population), or research and inquiry are crushed by the force of mass marketing, leaving us feeling foolish if we hesitate to accept the safety and value of the product or procedure.

You must do your own investigating. You must also resist the lull and coercion of marketing. Decades ago, it was print advertising, aimed at the public, with photos of pregnant celebrities like Lucille Ball endorsing a brand of cigarettes, or pharmaceutical company promotions to physicians, depicting a beautiful, healthy baby next to the copy:

"Really?" Yes... desPlex® (DES) *to prevent ABORTION, MISCARRIAGE and PREMATURE LABOR recommended for routine prophylaxis in ALL pregnancies.*

Today it is the phenomenon of prescription drug ads on TV. Same concept, yet in a different, more excessive and intensified form. Despite the quick babble of numerous, possible risk factors (including death in many of them) at the end of the commercial, the assumption of absolute benefit and safety is the objective.

I want you to be aware. It is imperative that you are aware. How many women who smoked throughout their pregnancies, and were exposed to pelvic x-rays, how many women who took DES and Thalidomide regretted not knowing about the research that existed, and heedlessly submitted to recommendations without debate? Use your intuition, dig for information, balance pros and cons, and proceed with caution, as you decide for yourself whether or not to take a pill or accept any therapeutic measure, no matter how many people in your life ridicule you and roll their eyes at your vigilance.

EDUCATION IN PRACTICE

Maybe you know someone who had the experience of giving birth without any real knowledge of or ability to advocate for their choices, yet everything still turned out just as they had hoped. Maybe *everyone* you know had that experience. So, why, oh why, can't you just sit back, not stress over learning about inductions and episiotomies, and purely focus on the fun things, like gender reveals and baby showers? It is absolutely true that all may still go well if you remain ignorant, as it actually did for me with my first two births. I guess the question is, under what circumstances and in which particular life experiences are you willing to take chances? When is it acceptable to you, personally, to do nothing but hope for the best? Safe, healthy outcomes in birth do occur *in spite* of what is done or not done, just as most people who ride a motorcycle without a

I suppose that the reason someone who would spend hours upon hours researching and choosing a car seat for their baby, but wouldn't give childbirth education a second thought, is that they are aware they have choices with varying consequences when it comes to baby equipment, but they aren't aware that they have choices with varying consequences when it comes to giving birth.

helmet are probably going to be just fine when they reach their destination. I suppose that the reason someone who would spend hours upon hours researching and choosing a car seat for their baby, but wouldn't give childbirth education a second thought, is that they are aware they have choices with varying consequences when it comes to baby equipment, but they aren't aware that they have choices with varying consequences when it comes to giving birth.

Now you have awareness. You've scraped the tip of the iceberg of consciousness in just a few pages of a book that some force of nature - some law of attraction - conspired to put in your hands. You may only be at the beginning stages of wading in the waters of understanding, but I bet you can begin to see the value in safe and healthy outcomes *because of,* not *in spite of* what you do or don't do. At times it may simply come down to probability, yet it's so much more than that. It's the wonder of empowerment, the most transcendent prize, which can only be attained when you are proactively learning and putting your knowledge into action. If your objective is to be empowered, if you do not plan on resigning yourself to an outcome determined by forces outside of your control, then you must educate yourself.

> *It's the wonder of empowerment, the most transcendent prize, which can only be attained when you are proactively learning and putting your knowledge into action.*

I encourage you to find the class or coach or system that works best for you. If you choose a class, make sure it is independently taught (as opposed to a hospital-based class), which removes the possibility of restrictions to the content, due to hidden agendas. You want to make sure you're receiving irrefutable, gold-standard, evidence-based information. Classes are most effective when they are structured around your needs, not the perspective of the educator. Teachers are facilitators. They are not authorities. They need to be coming from a place of empathy and honoring you as the expert on yourself. Look for a coach, not just an instructor. There should always be a healthy marriage between *respect* for your choices (the default) and *challenging* your choices through new information.

Logistically, from a scheduling angle, find a process that decreases your stress, not one that makes you more anxious. Most of the time, this distinction will be found in the level of flexibility being offered. Along with life's typical challenges, preparing to have a baby can add a new dimension of overwhelm. If you are an overachiever, first let me say, "I feel you", and then allow me to give you permission to stop the madness right now! I know I've been emphasizing the vital component of knowledge and preparation, but you don't have to read every article, research paper and book, and you might want to reconsider signing up for multiple classes. Here is yet one of many opportunities, as you prepare for your transition into parenthood, or your entrance into the further expansion of your family, to learn the art of balance. What you might gain from taking advantage of every possible option, you will lose in both physical and mental exhaustion.

Be aware that in the same vein of lack of individuality previously discussed, birth classes can also tend towards uniformity. If you're searching for the right "method" of childbirth education, factor in the certainty that your birth will be unique in every way. Just as there cannot be one correct way or one best way to reach a weight loss goal or to find optimal health overall, there is no one correct or best way to prepare for, or actually give birth. Considerations, such as possible medical conditions and physical limitations are obvious examples of how and why each person's experience needs to be treated individually. Less obvious, but of equal significance are things like clinical anxiety, past trauma, relationships, and various other circumstances.

Each method may bring something specific to the table, but there is no secret sauce to managing labor and birth. Childbirth education should be holistic (all-inclusive and thorough), touching on the process of knowing and tuning into your pregnant body, how to make connections between physical sensations and physiological changes that indicate progress during labor, natural comfort measures that contain no risk, and the full scope of medical interventions. If you're learning alongside your partner and/or anyone who will be present at your birth, an emphasis on physical and emotional support techniques is not only crucial for you, as the recipient of that support, but for them and their ability to stay present and calm, and to be as effective as possible. Additionally, information and ideas that can contribute to your health and the health of your baby during pregnancy would be beneficial, as would instruction on the topics of the first few hours in your newborn's life, and breastfeeding. You should complete a course of instruction on knowing how to make decisions as your labor unfolds and feeling prepared and confident throughout.

You might be attracted to testimonials of those who claim that one particular miraculous technique was the trick to a fairly effortless labor. Be careful with your fragile hopes. The reality is that you cannot manipulate every aspect of your response to labor with a single approach. My intention is not to disparage any particular program. In fact, I believe that learning a combination of strategies in an integrative way is ideal. You should learn the details of many choices that you can draw upon as you see fit. I'm simply cautioning you against maintaining unrealistic expectations.

Childbirth education should also be a means of facilitating your transition into parenthood. Becoming a mother is filled with uncertainty for most women. For those of you who already know you want to take classes, your chief expectation might be heavily centered on this turning point, even more than getting equipped for birth. Here's the really awesome part of the deeper aspects of childbirth education – the part that strengthens your belief in yourself, your confidence, and your communication skills: Once you put all of this into play and you build your self-efficacy through birth, this will now become a part of your personal history that you can draw upon as a new mother and as your baby grows up. You've undoubtedly experienced this before, in times when you accomplished or overcame something that you eventually, at some point in the future, used as a resource of pride and strength - a resource that caused you to feel capable. Childbirth education can shape your confidence and readiness for motherhood in that manner. Rather than through a step-by-step process, with distinct instructions, this education offers the hugely profound, unintended result of comprehensively preparing for birth.

THE LONG AND SHORT OF IT

Here's the summarized trickle-down effect illustrating the risk of birth-ignorance:

If you don't know your body, you don't know what's happening to your body, and if you don't know what's happening to your body, you are much more likely to be anxious, fearful, and stressed.

If you are anxious, fearful, and stressed, in combination with being oblivious to your options, you won't be able to manage pain or facilitate progress. Your anxiety will negatively affect your baby and your labor, causing more pain and anxiety, which can possibly lead to the need for medical interventions that might not have been necessary.

If you end up with otherwise unnecessary medical Interventions, you are stirring up a whole bunch of risk without benefit, for you and your baby.

Ignorance is not bliss. Ignorance is passive, while bliss is active. You "remain" ignorant, but you "find" bliss. You have to *do* something to reach that level of joy and fulfillment. When you're ignorant, you might be content and comfortable, like the feeling you get when you've just plopped down on the couch after a long day, zoned out in front of the TV, mindlessly eating a bowl of ice cream. It may seem pleasurable in the moment, but you're not exactly achieving any enduring, influential gratification and, most of the time, there will be negative consequences.

Learning, on the other hand, is part of the human experience, inherent in your natural state of being. Being open to new lessons enriches you, and it will certainly enrich the most important moments of your life, like birth. When you know better, you can do better, and then you can become better, for yourself and everyone in your world. Sorting through truths and myths leads to light bulb moments. These little, and sometimes big shifts affect the way you think about birth; the way you think about and plan for *your* birth. This is the jumping-off point for establishing your personal visions and dreams. Having the ability to distinguish between fact and fiction will prompt you to question, which in turn, will lead you down the path you're supposed to be on – the unknown path that seems so scary, many will not even venture a step. They will stay stuck being unknowing in the land of the unknown. But that will not be you, birth-informed goddess!

WHAT NOW?

○ Think – don't just act. Ask questions. Use your intuition.

○ Find an independently taught childbirth class and other forms of education that deliver evidence-based information and suit your personal needs and desires.

○ Break away from the masses who are birth-ignorant and those who don't honor birth as a holistic experience. Surround yourself with those who are truly birth-knowledgeable and who honor birth.

Thoughts and Actions

Chapter 3

DEAR SKEPTICAL PARTNER

"Blind belief in authority is the greatest enemy of truth."
- ALBERT EINSTEIN

O pen your mind, dear skeptical partner. I'm coming in.

Let's chat for a moment. You can trust me. I'm married to one of you. You're one part suspicious, one part resigned. You don't understand why things can't be left well enough alone, why we all can't just have faith in the way things are and be content. You wish you would stop being asked to "watch this, and read that", knowing there's probably some behind-the-scenes brainwashing going on by friends who grow their own sprouts. You're not jumping on some woo-woo bandwagon, agreeing to midwives and doulas and water births. No way are you compromising safety for some new-age experience. That crap is the opposite of science, the opposite of medicine – and you're not having any of it. You don't live in a hut on a mountain without indoor plumbing. You can't fathom why anyone in a first world country would choose to have a baby as if they did.

I understand and admire the intention. You just want everything to go well. You want whatever is best and safest for the person you love and for your baby. You're not looking to rock the boat, and you're certainly not feeling like it's going to do anyone any good to start experimenting with something other than what's tried and true.

You are not alone. What I mean by that is, not only are you in good company when it comes to your desire for excellent care, you are also not the only one who has been the victim of deep-rooted belief systems influenced by external forces. We are wired to be swayed by, to accept, and to internalize popular philosophies. With your new identity, as you embark on the birth of your child and the path of parenting, you're going to want to hold the reins of your established doctrine even tighter. I get it. But that is simply because you don't know what you don't know, and because all of that conditioning to keep the boat steady and not make waves has deep roots.

Many have expressed to me that their frame of reference around birth has always been that it was a medical procedure – that, just as if when you got sick you would go to the doctor and do whatever the doctor told you to do, you would, without question, follow their protocol for birth as well. Add to that the underlying fear that something could go terribly wrong if you don't go along with their policies and plan, and you're left with a complete lack of critical thinking when it comes to decisions in which medical care is involved. The pervasive thought process is, "Who am I to contradict the expert? On what basis do I have the right to do so?"

Others have harbored misconceptions of the less popular options for childbirth, rejecting choices like midwives for medical care, doulas for professional support, and water births. As one expecting dad put it, "I got hung up on the term 'midwives'

> *The pervasive thought process is, "Who am I to contradict the expert? On what basis do I have the right to do so?"*

because I thought of them like something from history, from antiquity, like that's how they used to do it in the Victorian era. So to say now, in our modern era, that you're going to have a midwife deliver your baby – all I could think of was that some woman was coming to your house and there would be crystals and chanting involved. It was the opposite of science, the opposite of medicine."

Of the scores of partners I've been acquainted with, the pushback is also around forsaking technology to any extent. It seems mad and irresponsible to abandon the miracle of present-day technology, especially in relation to anything medical, and particularly with regard to birthing a baby.

The biggest problem with all of these thoughts is that they're based solely on conjecture. As Marie Forleo, marketing and lifestyle expert, and bestselling author, terms it in her book, *Everything is Figureoutable,* these are "hand me down beliefs". Never once have you investigated and challenged these beliefs. I know that because, if you did, your unquestionable assertions would surely start to unravel.

So, now that I know your mind is a bit more open (which I've concluded because I began this chapter with that appeal, and because you're still reading) I think it's time to filter in some new ideas grounded in evidence-based information I'll bet you're not aware of. It's time to loosen those reins for the very reason you've been digging your heels in up until now... because we're talking about the most important thing in your life.

POP QUIZ FOR PARTNERS (OR ANYONE)

Let's see what you know and what you don't know and allow me to confer some accurate information right here.

What do you think?

> **Truth or Myth:** *You should make sure to get to the hospital quickly once your partner's water breaks because this means labor has started and the baby could come any second. There is also a high risk of infection after just a short period of time of ruptured membranes without contractions.*

This is folklore of the contemporary kind. In every movie and TV show where there is a pregnant character that will give birth sometime before the story ends, her water breaks, she freaks out, and immediately races to the hospital in lightning speed. Every. Single. One. *Sex in the City, Baby Mama, Friends.* In light of this prevailing stereotype, I understand why you might be confused. "This is all true!" you say, "I saw it on *Modern Family!*" You've been conditioned to believe that water breaking equals emergency. In *Fools Rush In* not only does Isabel's water break, but she screams at Alex to call 911.

Here's the deal: According to research cited in an Evidence Based Birth® Signature Article, titled: *Evidence on: Premature Rupture of Membranes,* "Estimates vary, but researchers say that about 8-10%, or 1 in 10 people, will have their water break before the onset of labor (Gunn et al., 1970)."

This is the first reason why the above statement is a myth. The odds that a pregnant woman's water will break before she begins having contractions are relatively small. The second reason is simply that babies don't just fall out. There's a lot of work to be done by a birthing woman's body, and a lot of work the baby needs to do to maneuver through the pelvis and birth canal. Therefore, rushing to the hospital is not necessary. Finally, it's important to examine whether or not there is actually a crisis that needs to be averted. The belief that ruptured membranes are immediate cause for concern with regard to the baby's well-being, is also inaccurate and misleading. If certain precautions are followed, such as avoiding numerous vaginal exams (something that only occurs when you get to the hospital as it is), evidence supports waiting for labor to begin on its own for up to 2-3 days, although even the most liberal care providers might have you come in a bit sooner. If the amniotic fluid is clear, and there are no complications that would otherwise cause you to rush to the hospital, stay comfortable, in your home. Wait for contractions to start, keep in touch with your care provider, and be the most indulgent, tender, reassuring and encouraging partner you can be.

Let's try another one:

Truth or Myth: *It is safer to monitor the baby continuously during labor, using an Electronic Fetal Monitor (EFM), the machine that picks up and records your baby's heart rate* *along with contractions, as opposed to intermittently applying a hand-held tool (like the Doppler used during prenatal visits), because the EFM is much more advanced and sophisticated, and because anything can happen at any time, so you don't want to go through labor without keeping the monitor on. You don't want to take a chance on missing something.*

I know you so badly want to believe that this is true because, after all, it refers to divine technology. But, alas, it too is a myth. If you think it's wise to follow science, research and evidence, as opposed to common theories that seem to make sense, you might be interested in the following scientifically established points.

It is appropriate to monitor a baby (fetus) continuously, if there is a high-risk situation, or if there are other interventions like an epidural (a regional anesthetic) or pitocin (a synthetic hormone to induce or augment contractions) being used. The Electronic Fetal Monitor is practical in these cases, as it would be unreasonable to expect nurses to spend hours with one birthing woman, constantly holding the device.

In low-risk labors, however, research shows that EFM is not beneficial to fetal health or outcome. There are no decreases in cerebral palsy, admissions to the neonatal intensive care unit, or fetal death. In other words, just because the technology is appealing, and it seems like it would have a great impact on increasing safety and decreasing risks – not to mention the fact that practically all laboring women giving birth in a hospital have the EFM as part of their birthing experience - it is not evidence-based. It is not doing what it was intended to do.

To add insult to injury, continuous EFM has been shown to increase the rate of Cesarean section. Why would that be? Why would you end up with a statistically significant increase in C-sections with the use of continuous Electronic Fetal Monitoring? Here are some reasons:

- There is reduced mobility for the laboring person because they must remain still in bed so that the weighted transducers stay in place on their large, round belly. This can cause:
  - an inability to use gravity and change positions.
  - great difficulty in managing the pain of labor, as the freedom to move and assume different positions is a major source of comfort.

  When the person in labor works with their body to encourage dilation of the cervix and the rotation and descent of the baby, the natural process of birth can take place. Without the ability to move and change positions, more medical interventions will likely be needed, either because of the decrease or cessation in labor progress, or because of the need for pain medication or an epidural. Each intervention has its set of risks, which can start the snowball effect toward an eventual C-section.

- Flawed interpretation of the data:
  - The technology may be state-of-the-art, but the findings are still subject to imperfect, and sometimes fallible human interpretation.

- Fear of litigation and a malpractice lawsuit:
  - It is much more common for a court of law to find in favor of the physician and hospital if an EFM

tracing is presented as proof of "unreassuring" fetal heart tones, where a subsequent C-section took place - as opposed to a case where there was no tracing, and it was determined that a C-section was not the best course of action. This can cause more doctors to, consciously or subconsciously, err on the side of legal caution, and perform C-sections with unwarranted ease.

One more:

> **Truth or Myth:** *A Certified Nurse Midwife provides the same medical care for an uncomplicated, low-risk pregnancy and birth that an Ob/Gyn does. The main distinction is that midwives are not trained surgeons.*

Truth! There are different types of training for midwives, each with their pros and cons, attracting various considerations around the profession – no one necessarily better or worse. Midwives who can work with all women, regardless of where they're giving birth (which is only dependent on their personal preferences) are Certified Nurse Midwives, and in some states, Certified Midwives. CNM's and CM's are highly skilled and trained medical professionals, providing pre and postnatal medical care in hospitals, prescribing and sometimes administering all screenings and procedures that doctors do. The main distinction is that they are not surgeons and cannot perform C-sections. Stay tuned for more details in Chapter 4.

These are only a few examples in which you may find that gaining further information discredits your entrenched assumptions. My hope is that the revelation you have experienced, causes you to start questioning and digging and finding more ways to distinguish between truths and myths. Begin to dissolve your stubborn defense of what you think the process should be, as you realize that some, if not all of your beliefs have no backing and the arguments are weak. If you are genuinely seeking the best care with the highest level of safety, it's important to know that there are many choices, and that Mother Nature rivals technology. It is imperative that you go in pursuit of the accurate information and valid options, so that you can be a true partner in creating your personal plan, and actually fulfill the desire to secure the best and safest birth experience for your partner and your baby.

At the very least, I'm urging a shift in mindset. The partner quoted earlier went on to say:

"I was shocked to actually go meet the midwives and see them in their white coats, carrying stethoscopes, in a facility that was just as modern and clean and sophisticated as any doctor's office."

As another partner declared, after being asked his thoughts on episiotomies (a surgical cut at the opening of the vagina):

"I had heard so many times about episiotomies, that doctors just did them because that's what they always do. They have to make a cut so it's easier for the woman to deliver. And then I found out it was totally misleading and mostly false. Once you get the information and you know the science behind it, it's abundantly clear that that's not how it's supposed to be. It's the opposite of how it's marketed or disseminated to the expecting parents who just nod up and down 'yes, yes, yes'."

IT'S WORTH THE WORK

You might be thinking, "I understand now that not everything is legitimately the way it seems. Maybe we shouldn't just assume that the common way is the safest, best way." Despite this, you're not completely convinced that spending the time and effort to take the next steps and do more than simply being on board with whatever your partner wants is worthwhile. The idea of confronting doctors and other medical professionals feels so uncomfortable and daunting. You may believe you only have the right to some peripheral involvement – that it's not really your place to be speaking up about any of this, even if the facts are compelling – because you're not the one carrying the baby and won't be the one giving birth. On top of that, you have way too much on your plate, between working and getting the baby's room ready, to be reading and taking classes, and frankly, it's overwhelming and not really your thing. It would be so much easier to just let this unfold and take your chances because, most of the time, everything turns out fine. I mean, the baby's coming no matter what, right? How much of a difference is it really going to make if you choose one thing over another, especially since, at the end of the day, you'll be relegated to a corner while everyone else around you takes over?

In part, you're still making assumptions. You don't think you have any control, and you're not assessing just how valuable this work is. Never forget this - You have a CHOICE as to what you ask for and receive, but to make an informed choice you have to be just that - informed. To put it in perspective for you, ask yourself how many hours you have spent researching the safety options, price points, and alternatives for buying a new family car. Now, compare that to the time you spent researching the safety options, support techniques, and possibilities for the birth of your child. I'm guessing there's a disparity, but don't be disheartened. There is still time to close the gap, and it is worth the work. With this kind of effort, you will be a strong and highly consequential presence during the birth of your baby.

Summon up the desire to learn what you need to learn to form an opinion about what is best for *you*, as the co-parent of your baby, the chief support person for your love, and the protector of the experience, in all ways.

To put it in perspective for you, ask yourself how many hours you have spent researching the safety options, price points, and alternatives for buying a new family car. Now, compare that to the time you spent researching the safety options, support techniques, and possibilities for the birth of your child.

Now that I've exposed you to examples of established myths, and you've gotten a taste of how those powerful, cultural messages are keeping you from tapping into the truth, I can't imagine you're not starting to think, "What more don't I know?"

Master this subject of preparing for birth so that you can be right there, on the front lines, with the plan that the two of you devised together. As you see yourself confidently communicating with your birth team, safeguarding your plan, and watching this experience manifest the way you had discussed, you might just feel like one partner who said, "We had this game plan, we went into the birthing room, and it was like winning the Super Bowl." I expect that even if things don't go exactly to plan, and you don't actually end up "winning", you're going to gain massive fortitude just by being in the game.

It's time to stop leaving well enough alone because that's what was modeled for you your whole life. Get the information and then evaluate the information. Be a communicator. Ask questions. Get involved. Form an opinion and gain the confidence it takes to interact with the people you hired, the ones who are getting paid to provide you with a monumental service. If you don't feel comfortable with their suggestions, ask for other options. If you feel pressured by an agenda that does not fit yours, gain the ability to provide an educated response. Of course, it would be great for you to learn physical techniques that would alleviate your partner's pain, but your ability to articulate and advocate is going to be just as, if not more important during the vulnerable, and sometimes, tumultuous moments of this birth experience. You can, and should, challenge decisions that are being made without your input. Not to get all psycho-babble on you, but what deep-rooted, unreasonable reverence for medical professionals are you harboring? In what other interactions in your role as a consumer do you feel you can't defend your belief that you know what is best for you, or question an expert after doing your homework?

You are entitled to respect, and you want to feel strong in a protector role, not sheepishly follow the rules like an insignificant little kid. You teach people how to treat you. The less you know, the more frightened you are, and the more you express the desire to be taken care of, the more likely it is that you will essentially be handing over your control. It's like you're saying, "Help her, I have no idea what to do". In that case, you will be pushed aside, not necessarily because the medical staff are rude, but because you're subliminally or overtly asking for them to take over – which is their specialty. They're typically not trained to put the power back in your hands, so if their first line of duty is to take over, and you're emphasizing that by being meek and afraid and unknowledgeable (as opposed to asking questions and helping in the advocacy process), then you will further entrench the attitude that this is purely a medical event for which you are not skilled. This is not purely a medical event. Often times it's not a medical event at all. And with knowledge, you are absolutely skilled.

I also don't want you to miss out on the amazing opportunity to forge a deeper bond with the mother of your child through this process. Stop. Think. What are we talking about here? Bringing your baby into this world is most definitely *the* opportunity to shape a powerful union.

Please, please, *please*, be open to learning because in the context of doing so, you will get to know each other in such a deep way, like never before. Peel back the layers together – yes, of data and research, but more profoundly, of your longings for this experience. Walk through every part of the planning consciously, learning more and more about your motivations behind those longings. Have opinions. Have wants. See each other in a new and different and thrilling way. For yourself and for your relationship, gain the ability to arrive at this place, so eloquently recounted from one partner's experience: "I find myself saying, 'I made it through that. I did that'. That ability to do something you didn't think you could, can translate into being able to do other things that you're hesitant to do, or nervous about."

Then there's your unique transformational experience of becoming a parent, and the distinct emotion, including fear and excitement, you will have around that. Being an integral part of the birth process sets you up for a confidence that cannot be achieved in any other way.

WHAT I HOPE YOU WILL SAY TO OTHER PARTNERS SOME DAY

Before I wrap up our time together here, dear partner, in the hope that you are a little less skeptical and more inquisitive as a result of our time together, I want to leave you with some words my own always-skeptical-but-also-enlightened husband shared with me.

"You can have a great birth experience either way, knowing or not knowing, but to be informed on something that's so important, the most important thing in your life, seems non-negotiable to me. I say this all the time - people spend more time investing in a vacation or a car, than they do things that really matter. And this really matters. So why wouldn't you roll up your sleeves, get involved, understand the pros and cons, understand the information, and then you and your partner can come to a sensible decision, based on facts and not hearsay?

It's like the example of trying to learn golf when I was growing up. My father would always say, keep your head down and your left arm straight. I don't know where he got it from, but it seemed like that was the teaching method. And then when I went to a professional and I got some lessons and I told him that, he said, 'Where'd you get that from? That's utter bullshit. You don't want to keep your head down. You don't want to keep your left arm straight.' And so, you know, people believe what they hear all the time without questioning it. So I should have said back then, 'Why do I keep my head down? And why do I keep my left arm straight? And then I could decide what I wanted to do based on that information. Should I continue that way or not? Is there a better method?"

He might be reluctant and doubtful, just like you, but he's also a pretty insightful dude. You might want to listen to him.

WHAT NOW?

○ Talk to your partner – the woman you love who is carrying your baby. Ask her what her thoughts are about this pregnancy and upcoming birth. What is it that she wants most – from you and from this experience? Be vulnerable, open, and honest about your own feelings, hesitations and fears.

○ Get educated. Don't make assumptions. Flesh out the facts. Ask questions, and then ask *more* questions. Find the answers that help you to feel confident in your decision-making, and comfortable with your choices. Don't leave anything to chance.

○ Seek to combine a mix of evidence and emotions, in alliance with your partner, when sorting through the options that will create your personal, ultimate birth experience.

○ Consider all the things you've scrutinized in your life – the things that you valued the most – where the outcome of the action, the purchase, the decision was critical. A chosen career path, a house, a marriage. Your attitude wasn't: whatever will be will be; if everyone else is doing it like that, it must be the best way; it's too overwhelming to research and plan, or too risky to set a goal and follow through. This is the *birth of your baby*, the birth of your family. There is nothing more important. Contemplate all angles. Every option. Scrutinize as much as possible.

Thoughts and Actions

_____

_____

_____

_____

_____

_____

_____

_____

_____

_____

_____

_____

_____

_____

Chapter 4

BIRTH IS A TEAM SPORT

"Collaboration is the essence of life.
The wind, bees and flowers work together, to spread
the pollen."

- AMIT RAY

My third and last pregnancy took place 12 years before my husband decided to sign up for his first full Ironman triathlon. During the planning of that birth, I could not have known how many analogies I would, one day, make to the planning of this triathlon. Just as he would be preparing his body and mind for crossing a finish line, I had prepared my body and mind for giving birth. Just as he would eventually execute a list of details (goggles, wetsuit, bike, pump), I had checked off my own list (birth ball, washcloths, music, candles). In the same way he would need a team of people providing their individual skill sets and strengths to make sure he was properly trained and supported for the Herculean event of the triathlon, I too had needed a collaborative team for the colossal event of birth.

A birth team consists mostly of people who will support you in some way during labor, but there are other team members who will or may be part of the prenatal and postpartum periods: midwives, doctors, doulas, nurses, lactation consultants, fitness and nutrition specialists, photographers, pelvic floor therapists, mental health counselors, family and friends. Each person on your birth team will bring something to the table. With the new information you receive as you become more and more educated throughout your pregnancy, you'll want to set personal goals in the way of preferences and expectations. Working with the right team will increase the likelihood of achieving those goals.

Like going to a spa where you have interactions with a variety of skilled professionals, working, either one at a time or simultaneously, to tend to and pamper you, your birth team is tuned into your desires and your needs, and the needs of your baby. Each of their strengths is focused on fulfilling your requests, intuitively tapping into what you may find helpful in the moment and overall, and, for medical providers, keeping a watchful eye on any deviation from what is considered to be normal.

It is very easy to slip into a place of fear, confusion, and self-doubt when your labor is not progressing as envisioned, and when you are exhausted and in pain. When things don't go as planned (which is always, to some degree), partnering with those who are committed to your vision, and can help you to shift while still maintaining control, can keep you on track. As you are focusing on contractions, they can offer new ideas, suggestions, and ways to level up the support you will need.

Your partner also does not have to feel entirely alone and responsible for providing continuous support, encouragement, and reassurance, especially when they will need those three things for themselves.

When things don't go as planned (which is always, to some degree), partnering with those who are committed to your vision, and can help you to shift while still maintaining control, can keep you on track.

This idea may seem odd to you. You may never have thought about assembling a team in light of the fact that the prevailing mindset is - everything around birth will be done for you, including the gathering of those that are supposed to be there.

You chose your doctor, or at least the practice as a whole, and you have your partner. Why would you want anyone else? It's not like you're planning an event where you need to consult with and include a bunch of people.

Ah, but wait a second – actually, you are indeed planning such an event. Although different in many ways from a party or fundraiser or holiday gathering, giving birth should be high on your list of the most important events of your life. In order to secure the best experience for this extraordinary celebration, I encourage you to think of it as just that – a celebration – one in which teamwork and collaboration are essential toward the outcome you hope for.

WHO AND HOW DO YOU CHOOSE?

Like everything else about your birth, this is personal and should be highly individualized. In the same way you shouldn't feel pressured into making the choices your best friend made, you also shouldn't be discouraged or prevented from having with you whomever you determine will be an asset in one way or another. Consider taking this metaphor as you approach the selection process: showing up to an Ironman triathlon with no coach, no one to cheer you on, check your bags and your bike, no trained volunteers manning the kayaks to secure your safety in the water, no one to direct you on the course or assist you in the aid stations, would be the stuff of triathlete nightmares. Showing up to your birth without the people who could increase your ability to secure the easiest, safest, most fulfilling birth experience possible might just be the stuff of *your* nightmares. Without even one of these people, you are potentially risking more difficulty, confusion, intimidation, insecurity, anxiety, suspicion, and regret. It's that vital.

Let's start with your medical providers.

Obstetricians and Midwives
Before choosing which primary medical provider you want for your pregnancy and birth, it would be helpful to know the differences between the two dominant options.

There is a general distinction in the fundamental philosophy between obstetrics and midwifery. Directly tied into what is taught during the training for each profession is, quite possibly, the most significant difference. It is the way in which birth is viewed. While obstetricians see birth as a medical event, as they are trained physicians and surgeons with a focus on the complications of

68

pregnancy and childbirth, midwives see birth as a physiological event, as they are trained care providers with a focus on normal pregnancy and childbirth. Obstetric care is generally high-tech, low-touch. Midwifery care is generally low-tech, high-touch.

Logistically speaking, prenatal appointments with obstetricians usually last a few minutes. During labor you may only see your doctor briefly once they arrive at the hospital, if they're not already there, and sometimes only when birth is imminent. Prenatal appointments with midwives are scheduled further apart to leave time for discussions and counseling, in addition to the standard physical examinations and screenings at each stage of pregnancy.

Midwives are skilled diagnosticians who address and treat complications, but their primary goal is to keep the care they provide woman-focused, consulting and educating on ways to maintain physical and mental health before, during and after your baby is born.

Midwives work with low-risk and high-risk pregnancies. Because there are a range of circumstances that would deem a pregnancy "high risk", and because it can be both mentally and medically disadvantageous to draw parallels between each condition, it's worth taking a moment to discuss this here, specifically as it relates to age. Pregnant women who are 35 and older are labeled "advanced maternal age" and automatically considered to be high risk. Although the vast majority who go to term will have healthy babies, evidence does show a slightly increased risk of stillbirth throughout pregnancy in older women than in younger women. However, care by an obstetrician, as opposed to a midwife, would not reduce those risks. In fact, based on research, those in this category who chose a midwifery-led model of care, were shown to have fewer interventions and excellent outcomes.

When obstetrical attention is needed (in times when complications are outside of the scope of midwifery) midwives can and will identify these complications and refer to an obstetrician. Depending on the situation, there can either be continuity of care, with collaboration between obstetrician and midwife, or the care can be entirely managed by the obstetrician. Only obstetricians can perform surgeries, including C-sections. Strictly on the physical end, and in relation to qualifications and capability, you can think of it like this: You visit your dentist to maintain your oral health - for cleanings and exams. They can also perform diagnostic tests, like X-rays, and treat an array of the most common issues, such as cavities, root canals and crowns. If they determine that you have gum disease, they may refer you to a periodontist, or if they ascertain that your pain is coming from impacted wisdom teeth, they would probably refer you to an oral surgeon. In both cases, you would, most likely, follow up and continue seeing your dentist in addition to the specialist.

My intention is always to provide information that will help you to make the decisions that are best for you. It is never to persuade you to make a particular choice, one way or another. Having said that, I must add a few facts about midwifery care here, as the ideas around midwives are still, widely, misunderstood.

- o Midwives can catch babies at home or in free-standing birth centers, but about 95% of Certified Nurse Midwife/Certified Midwife-attended births take place in hospitals.
- o Midwives do not only care for women who want natural births. They have the skills to facilitate that plan, offering physical and emotional support and guidance, but the primary objective is to provide what is needed and chosen

by the birthing woman, including epidurals and other forms of pain relief.

o   Midwifery care is not just pregnancy and birth care. Midwives provide primary care throughout a woman's life, including gynecological exams, screenings, vaccinations, family planning, fertility counseling and menopausal care.

It is still appropriate to work with an obstetrician from the start, and throughout a low-risk, uncomplicated pregnancy, even though midwifery care is more of the specialty in this area. Knowing the distinctions will help you come to your own personal conclusions as to what is best for you. Although I am laying out specific details to be used as a roadmap toward that decision, the choice you make should always be based on your perception around the relationship. With whom do you feel the most comfortable? With whom do you believe you'll receive the best clinical care, the highest level of holistic care, and the greatest chance of individualized care, in addition to respect for your autonomy? Don't just take the recommendation of a friend or from responses to a Facebook post, based solely on who they "like". Their reasons for liking this practitioner may not be in line with what is important to you in realizing your ultimate birth experience, even if they are recommending someone who has a good bedside manner. Their reasons for liking this practitioner may have only to do with how nice this person is. Believe me, being nice is important, but it will be meaningless if they are not practicing evidence-based, individualized care, and you end up stressing over whether or not you're going to have control and get the support you need during your labor.

Whether you choose to work with a midwife or an obstetrician, I want you to have a healthy attitude about the role they will play in your birth. Instead of regarding your caregivers as omnipotent divine beings, consider them as lifeguards. Swimming in the ocean rarely involves being saved. We wade into the water, knowing how to make our way through the waves, at some point diving into them, or just ducking under when we've passed the shallow end. Once we're far enough out, we navigate those waves and either bob around or swim until we decide to come out. Imagine if while doing your thing, the lifeguard decided to jump off his post, dash into the water, pull you out, and start CPR. No riptide. No potential drowning. No crisis to avert. He just assumed that this was part of the responsibilities he was trained to perform, and whether or not there was a need, in the moment, to actually perform them, he felt compelled to routinely apply his skills, for a number of personal, underlying reasons. You'd probably be pretty confused, not to mention pissed off. That's not to say you're not grateful for the lifeguard's presence on the high tower, as there actually could be a potentially unforeseen, dangerous situation, at which time you'd expect his help. But you know how to swim, just as you know how to give birth. As the lifeguard's expertise offers protection and assistance, should you need it, your medical practitioner's expertise does the same. If you don't need that assistance; if there's no need to rescue you, their chief role is to keep a watchful eye.

Instead of regarding your caregivers as omnipotent divine beings, consider them as lifeguards.

When it's appropriate to restructure part of the team

In professional baseball, when management feels the team is floundering and could be doing better, changes are made. Whether it's replacing a closer in the bottom of the ninth during a particular game or firing a manager and hiring a new one in the middle of a season, these decisions are made with unquestionable certainty. The fundamental motive driving every bit of strategy, both on the field and behind the scenes, is to strengthen the team and achieve the goal of winning games, and eventually, the World Series.

Your birth experience is the World Series, only much more extraordinary, momentous, significant and powerful. More earth-shaking and life-changing than any other game on Earth. If you believe anyone on your team is going to prevent you from achieving your goals, you must make a change. It is not easy to do this. But you must. It is vital to the process of actualizing all you have worked for. Without all team members being on board with your blueprint, the plan you put so much effort into creating, you are setting yourself up for failure.

"But", you may be wondering, "what about the labor and delivery nurses, who I don't get to choose? What if one or more are discouraging and disapproving and they are upsetting me?" This is definitely a solvable problem. Nurses, especially if you don't choose to engage with a doula, are your main sources of support once you arrive at the hospital. Although this too may seem difficult and antagonistic, you can, and should, absolutely request a different nurse when faced with confrontations that are sabotaging your intentions and your labor. It is always your call. If you feel that it's not a huge issue; that you're managing without their support, and it's not worth rocking the boat, then, by all means, let it go.

However, at any time you feel more tense when the nurse is in the room, or if you are being mocked and disrespected, or bullied in any way, you need to communicate this to the nurse manager, your doctor or midwife, and insist on a change.

I'll leave you with this reminder: You are an active consumer, not a passive patient.

Doulas

A labor doula is a trained professional who provides continuous physical, emotional, and informational support to a mother before, during and shortly after childbirth. Research shows decreases in the risk of Cesareans and medications for pain relief and increases in the overall satisfaction with the birth experience when support is given by a doula. In my own experiences, being the recipient of doula support and being the doula *giving* support to others, I have witnessed palpable decreases in anxiety, and increases in confidence and the ability to advocate. A doula does not usurp the role of the partner as loving "coach". She does not take over, but rather, supports the partner, offering suggestions for comfort measures that he or she can employ alone or together, alongside her. Partners are more enthusiastic and at ease because they are receiving the reassurance they need in order to provide that same reassurance in their role as "coach". They tend to relax into this role when the duties are shared, when they no longer feel that they have to know everything and remember everything, and when they have a professional by their side.

Doulas will assist you in acquiring knowledge and will encourage you to use your right to informed consent. When a recommendation is made by a medical provider during labor, they may ask you if you understand the recommendation, if you have questions and if you need more information. Doulas are not clinicians. They do not perform vaginal exams or any other medical procedures. They don't check blood pressure, temperature, or fetal heart tones, and they don't administer medication.

Some people are under the impression that if they have a doula with them during their labor and birth, the doula will relieve them of some of their responsibility to advocate for themselves. They believe that she will stand up for them, fight for what they want, and defend their choices. That is, in fact, outside of their scope of responsibility, and can, justifiably, get them kicked out of the labor room. Although a doula might direct certain thoughts and questions to the medical staff as part of the birth team, she will not communicate for you, or advocate for what you want on your behalf. She will encourage you to express your own, personal needs, preferences and concerns, and she will help you to do so.

Partners are often concerned that inviting a doula onto the team will take away from the intimacy of the birth experience. I want to assure you that, with everyone on the team acting professionally, giving you the benefit of their very best skills while staying in their lane, the entire experience will be enhanced. In many ways, the doula will protect your privacy and improve your sense of connectedness.

On one occasion I was a doula for a couple who had the goal of a natural birth, without medical intervention. Even though there were no complications, the labor progress was very slow and prolonged. The couple tried many techniques and utilized many comfort measures, but exhaustion was beginning to overpower the effectiveness of the contractions. Their doctor suggested pitocin as a way to augment labor. Because pitocin can cause contractions that feel stronger and more painful, and often come at closer intervals than those that are naturally occurring, he also recommended that she get an epidural to manage the increased pain he assumed she would experience once the pitocin kicked in. She agreed to the pitocin but did not want the epidural. This was a personal choice, made with the consideration of the benefits and risks involved; a choice not everyone would make, and, apparently, a choice her doctor was not used to his patients making in similar situations. It definitely was not the choice he wanted them to make, as he became more and more agitated while trying to convince them that this is how it should be done. When they stated that they felt they wanted to try the pitocin first, and wait to see if she could manage, what they hoped would be just a short while of strong contractions because she was very close to being able to push, his frustration began to feel menacing. At that point, after observing and allowing this couple to do their own communicating, I saw that they were becoming visibly intimidated and beaten down. I calmly asked them if they would like some time alone to discuss their options, and suggested that we all (her mother, the nurse, and the doctor) step out into the hallway for a few minutes. The doctor did so begrudgingly and then, once outside, proceeded to demand that I tell them to get the epidural. Although feeling somewhat bullied myself, I firmly explained that it was not my role, as a doula, to talk a client *into* or *out of* anything. I needed to be clear that my place on the team was completely separate from the doctor – that I did not work for him and I did not have an allegiance to support his wishes, whether I was in agreement with them or not. Once we re-entered the room, their ability to defend their decision was strong and resolute. The pitocin got her over the hump, she worked with her body to manage the painful contractions without the epidural, and within the hour, she gave birth safely and on her own terms.

If you're considering including a doula on your birth team, do your research, ask lots of questions to both friends who might have hired a doula for their births, and doulas themselves. Ask about their services, what they do and what they don't do, and get a feel for whether this is someone you like and trust and want to have with you at your birth.

Family and Friends
During the planning of my third birth, I had complete control over who would be part of my team, as this birth would take place in my home. With this flexibility, I was able to include the people that would each have a unique role, without any restrictions.

I had been working with a midwife, who was affiliated with a major university hospital. She was at the helm of my medical care. I also invited my two mentors to be with me, one as my doula (and videographer!) and one, who was on her path to becoming a midwife, as my midwife's assistant. My husband was my source of loving support and was also an excellent co-doula. Those four team members provided me with the perfect mix of care and support.

In addition, I also chose to prepare my two older children, who, at the time, were six and four years old, to be part of the experience. They were never pressured to participate, or even attend, if they decided not to at any point in time. In order to execute this plan, with its emotional and logistical uncertainties, I asked a special friend, who my children felt particularly comfortable with, to join us during labor to, first, play games with, and generally occupy the kids, and then to accompany them in my bedroom, where I would give birth.

In this mix there was one glaring exclusion. My mom. My whole life, up until that point, I was very close to my mother. She was my source of comfort in many ways, but she was also a worrier. If I had the sniffles, she would call several times a day to see how I was feeling, check up on my symptoms, and make sure it hadn't turned into something worse. She had been somewhat overprotective when I was a child and carried with her an underlying air of fear and foreboding, passed down from her mother, and probably, her mother before her. From an emotional place, I wanted my mom, who I loved dearly and who had instilled in me my joyful fascination with birth, to be in that room. She had been a part of this pregnancy, and all of my pregnancies, which deepened our connection and brought so much amazement and excitement to our relationship. I wanted her to have the rare and miraculous experience of watching her daughter give birth and her grandchild arrive earth-side. But I knew I could not have her there; not if I understood and valued what it would take to secure an environment conducive to a labor I could manage with confidence and peace. I knew that if my mom was there, she would be nervous. My possible loud moaning, as I worked through contractions, would further increase her anxiety, which would be palpable to me, as much as she would try to hide it. I realized that I could not take the chance of having any other experience than one in which I could be physically and mentally free to do what I needed to do to birth this baby.

Having this conversation with her, honestly revealing my feelings, and being in conflict with what I wished for but knew I couldn't have, was very difficult. But, at the end of the day, my mother was full of grace. There was nothing she would have done, no point she would have argued, if it hurt me in any way. Mothers are habitually wired to express that they only want what is best for their children,

BIRTH IS A TEAM SPORT

but we all know that there are natural, human, understandably self-serving characteristics that often hinder that intention. My mother was the exception. Not once in my life, to my recollection, did she do anything but what was best for her children, and this would be no more apparent than when I told her I couldn't have her with us at the birth of her "baby's" baby. She lived less than 15 minutes away, so we planned for her to come over as soon as possible once the baby was born - which she did, in the middle of the night, without the tiniest indication that this could have been anything but the most wonderful moment of her life.

This is my hope for you: that you will have the intuition and the strength to know yourself and your needs for your upcoming birth, that you will communicate those needs and request the support that will facilitate all of the components of your ultimate birth experience, even if that means holding space for the hurt feelings of people you love. Do not compromise.

Envision your birth. I know it's difficult to imagine what the circumstances will be and exactly how you'll feel, especially if this is your first birth, but you know yourself and how you typically manage situations that provoke some anxiety – ones in which you have had previous unsavory confrontations, or ones where you are on unchartered territory. If you know that

> *This is my hope for you: that you will have the intuition and the strength to know yourself and your needs for your upcoming birth, that you will communicate those needs and request the support that will facilitate all of the components of your ultimate birth experience, even if that means holding space for the hurt feelings of people you love.*

you need people on your team who are calm and reassuring and you fear your mom cannot be that person, as I did, then you must communicate clearly, well in advance of the day you go into labor. It is often helpful to include her in the classes you're taking or have her present during prenatal visits or meetings with your doula. I'm a fan of having someone else present – sort of like a mediator – when discussing sensitive subjects with those you care about. When emotions are high, it's easier to hear the full scope of intent if your initial thoughts are backed up with some rationale by someone who is not emotionally connected. The sting may still be there, but the news will be more easily digested. I wanted my mom to pause and look inside herself, so she would give a sincere answer when I asked her if she felt she could be calm and reassuring in the midst of a tense situation, if I was crying or roaring like a tigress to manage my contractions. I urged her to step outside of the fantasy, to see herself in those realistic moments and imagine how she might react.

Regardless of whether your family and friends, who you might need to have these tough conversations with, will react as my mother did, or with impulsive, raw emotion, you must hold your ground. Birth is not a spectator sport. Please don't invite people to your birth because you want to make them happy by honoring and gifting them with this experience. Invite people to your birth who you know will effectively support you. Take pictures and video if you want to share that moment with certain friends and family members. Invite them to be waiting close by (if that doesn't make you anxious) so that they can be included as soon as you are ready. But remember that you'll be working very hard during labor. As powerful and amazing as this time will be, it is not a party – at least not in the traditional sense. You have no obligation to anyone but yourself.

WHAT YOU MAY WANT AND WHAT YOU MAY NOT

In one mom's description of her birth, she told me: "All the people that attended my labor were extremely intuitive, skillful and loving. I trusted them during labor and birth and felt extremely secure and important." Putting the effort into assembling a team that can offer you their intuition, expertise, and loving care, a team that you trust, that considers you the leader of your experience, will position you to have a truly great birth.

If your efforts at assembling this team are crude, or you decide to leave this part entirely to chance, you could end up with a birth team you did not choose; with individuals who are not inclined to lift you up, who do not share your vision, and who are just doing their job. You could be surrounded by people who create stress, when one of your top goals should be to decrease stress. The fallout could easily be a cycle of increased pain, slowed progression, and more interventions. Don't miss out on the opportunity to be supported by individuals who, in collaboration, could influence the ease of your labor and help you to retain your control and feel less apprehensive and intimidated.

I once heard someone refer to their birth team as their "bubble". My interpretation of this is a world within a world, the place you choose to be, where you are not corrupted by the fear of others; the fear that is pervasive and can shift your own beliefs. Instead, you are surrounded by calm and reason, and people you trust who say things to you like, "It looks like you're having a big baby, and your body is perfectly capable of birthing a big baby" as opposed to, "It looks like you're having a big baby, so we're not going to *let* you wait for labor to start because if this baby gets any bigger you're going to need a c-section". It's the difference between, "Birth is normal. You can do this. How exciting!" and, "Birth is treacherous. You may not be able to do this. How frightening." The world in the bubble is not less competent, logical, or intellectual. Being hyper-vigilant is in no way better than being vigilant, and being hyper-vigilant and cynical absolutely does not decrease risk and increase safety. I say this because it is a common opinion that the lack of persistent worry and unrelenting apprehension defines someone who is unintellectual and featherbrained. So, for those who believe that the bubble is full of foolish and credulous nitwits, who are ignoring science in lieu of fairy dust, I assure you that is not the case. On the contrary, if you get that "bubble" feeling from the team you assembled through well-researched efforts, you will have a level of care that actually *does* increase your safety and decrease your risks, while bolstering your mental health, which is, in great part, a contributor to your ultimate birth experience.

WHAT NOW?

○ If you're not pregnant yet, now is the perfect time to set up consultation appointments with doctors and midwives. If you are currently pregnant but are not comfortable with the practice you have chosen (which can happen once you become knowledgeable and realize you're not aligned), this is also a good time to make those consultation appointments. Many practices will accept low-risk (and even some high-risk) cases toward the end of pregnancy.

○ I strongly recommend taking a childbirth class. They are not all equal in their curriculums and approaches, so take the time to speak with instructors and gather as much information as possible before making your decision.

○ Decide if you'd like to have a labor doula on your team. Create a list of questions and needs and review your list with at least two doulas/doula practices you are considering.

○ Look into starting a relationship with a lactation consultant. Yes, now. If you're planning to breastfeed, you want to have a connection to the person you can reach out to before you give birth.

○ In the same vein, explore hiring a postpartum doula for after your baby is born. The special skills of a postpartum doula will afford you the emotional, physical and informational support that is so critical in the days and weeks you are learning how to be a mom to an infant, while also needing to take care of yourself.

o Consider engaging with a pelvic floor therapist and other postpartum resources, including support groups and private mental health specialists who are uniquely skilled in the area of postpartum. This is an empowering step toward preparing for optimal health as you transition into motherhood. Creating these connections in advance can prevent any delays and pressures you'd encounter by scrambling to find these resources if your needs were to become urgent.

o Include family and friends by asking them to provide indirect support, if you choose not to have them with you during your labor and birth. Ask them if they would:
  • take care of pets and other children.
  • straighten up your house and throw in a load of laundry.
  • make sure there's food in the house for when you return (or for just before, during, and after a home birth).

Thoughts and Actions

_____

_____

_____

_____

_____

_____

_____

_____

_____

_____

_____

_____

_____

Chapter 5

SORTING THROUGH YOUR TOOLKIT

"I suppose it is tempting, if the only tool you have is a hammer, to treat everything as if it were a nail."
- ABRAHAM MASLOW

In our culture, where the influencers have created a climate of sameness, and those being influenced have accepted the canned version of birth, we've all but stopped searching for ways to improve our individual experiences. Most birthing women are completely unaware that they walk into labor with two "bags" – one that contains tools they can use to relieve pain and facilitate labor that don't include risk, and one with tools that are a means to the same end but do include risk. I call these the "Natural Bag" and the "Medical Bag". One is not better than the other. They are each valuable. Unfortunately, the bulk of the tools in the Natural

Bag are generally unfamiliar, and even the few commonly known medical tools are dispensed more than they are chosen. Women suffer through their labors until the point in which they can get an epidural. They welcome drugs to stimulate and accelerate contractions, at times oblivious to the simple steps they can take to work with their bodies.

The idea that it is impossible to control the labor and birth process is what may be stopping you from thinking a toolkit even exists, much less looking to learn what is in it. Although contractions are involuntary, everything you do or don't do during your labor can influence their effectiveness. You have a job. A big one. It is to work with the birth process; to support it and manage the pain and power it will, inevitably, bring.

Although the choice of where you plan to give birth precedes your labor, and is, therefore, not directly part of the toolkit contents, it is the first major option you will need to consider as you set yourself up for a smooth, safe, and joyful experience. In the Natural Bag, you'll be including your environment – the tools you'll use to create an atmosphere of calm and inspiration. But think about this: You can listen to ocean waves on your headphones, and diffuse essential oils while inside a haunted house, yet I'd bet these strategies would fall pretty short if your intention was to feel peaceful and focused in that particular physical space.

Where you choose to have your baby should be where you feel at ease and safe, which is not necessarily the same as where you are, in fact, safest. Here again lies a compelling reason why you need to first sort through all of the information, become aware of the evidence, and foster a personal view of birth that is not influenced by the popular view. Once you get to that place,

SORTING THROUGH YOUR TOOLKIT

whether it's a place you resided all along, or one that is new and unexpected, you can truly determine where you will, eventually, feel like you're in the *best* place. Evidence may be irrefutable, but a laboring woman's peace of mind will be a substantial factor in the outcome. As emphasized before, knowing the evidence is vital. However, just because research proves that a healthy woman having a normal pregnancy is just as safe, if not safer giving birth at home, a healthy woman having a normal pregnancy, who is informed, and after taking the time to weigh all the elements of her ultimate birth experience concludes that she will feel safe giving birth in a hospital, should give birth in a hospital. Continuous surges of adrenaline are not your friend in labor. Ask yourself these questions: "Will I feel more secure and able to work with my labor if there is an operating room down the hall, or will I feel safe and in control in a quiet, familiar space? Will I be more anxious with or without a large team of medical professionals and devices surrounding me?" The conclusions you come to are personal and will reveal the choice that is best for you.

The one point I want you to come away with here, in *all* of your choices, from every piece of information and guidance I am sharing with you on this topic and throughout this entire book, is that you are not being judged. I, personally, only care that you figure this all out for yourself once you have distinguished between fact and fiction, and you've made the effort to connect your personal truths to scientific truths. I don't think there's a right way and a wrong way, and neither should you, no matter how much of that inevitable judgment is being hurled at you. No comparisons. No competition. No guilt. This could not be more relevant than in our discussion about the venue in which you give birth. You may be part of a community of women who could not fathom planning their births in a hospital.

Just as the why and how of giving birth are yours and yours alone, where you determine is best for you should also always be validated and respected.

You may all feel that having your babies in birth centers or at home is absolutely the best choice. That doesn't make hospital births wrong, even if you determine they're wrong for you. The same is true if, in the end, you decide that you are, indeed, more at ease in a hospital. Just as the *why* and *how* of giving birth are yours and yours alone, *where* you determine is best for you should also always be validated and respected.

UNPACKING THE BAGS

This is far from a complete list of tools you have to choose from, but let's look at some of them.

Your Natural Bag

POSITIONS DURING LABOR

Movement during labor might just be your greatest asset, for it addresses both pain relief and progress. If you ask a woman who has gone through labor how it felt to have contractions while lying in bed, mostly reclined, and very still, she'll tell you it was extremely difficult. Without the reference of movement and position changes, she would probably be the woman who describes labor as excruciating. This doesn't mean that labor, with the benefit of movement, is a walk in the park. What is true, though, is that women are much more able to manage the pain of contractions if they are not remanded to bed and instructed to lay still for any number of reasons, the most common being to ensure an accurate recording of the baby's heart rate on the Electronic Fetal Monitor. It feels so much more natural and comfortable to stand and kneel; to lean and rock and sway while contractions are doing their thing.

If you weren't drawing upon media references of what birth is supposed to look like, if you weren't assuming you were supposed to lay in bed during labor, if no one was instructing you to keep your arms straight and your body in a fixed position, you would never choose to be this way. Your instincts, just like the instincts of any other mammal that isn't human, would be to move, or at least, periodically change into positions that eased discomfort and pain.

If you weren't drawing upon media references of what birth is supposed to look like, if you weren't assuming you were supposed to lay in bed during labor, if no one was instructing you to keep your arms straight and your body in a fixed position, you would never choose to be this way.

Likewise, various positions and movement will bring about progress. It is nature's design - her perfect plan. Besides the work your uterus is doing to open your cervix, it also needs to catalyze your baby's rotations and descent through your pelvis.

Effective positions for comfort and progress are usually some variation of being upright. Examples would include:

○ Standing while leaning into a wall or over a high surface
○ Standing and gently swaying in a slow dance movement with your partner or anyone supporting you

- ○ Walking/pacing
- ○ Hands and knees, on the floor or on the bed, rocking your hips side to side
- ○ Kneeling with your chest resting on a stack of pillows or a "birth ball" (a stability/exercise ball), rocking your hips side to side
- ○ Sitting on the ball, moving your lower body side to side, back and forth, and/or in a circular motion
- ○ Squatting on a birth stool or in bed, assisted by those supporting you, or with the use of a squatting bar that attaches to a hospital bed

Because the birth process can benefit from various positions and movement, and your ability to manage the pain of contractions may depend on this, it is imperative that you condition your body for the physical strength and stamina required. Think of the preparation you will put into your physical health and wellness before conceiving (if you have that option) and during pregnancy as the way in which you "sharpen" this amazing tool in your toolkit. Optimal nutrition, consistent exercise, healthy sleep habits, and de-stressing through meditation, mindfulness and other modalities, will prepare you for the ability to use this particular tool, and get the most out of it. Keep in mind that birth is a test of endurance, and the better shape you're in, physically and mentally, going into the "race", the better chance you have of reaching and excelling at your goals.

Be prepared and pay attention to your body as labor progresses. Listen – do not ignore or decide in advance which positions you absolutely will or will not take. Your body has such wisdom in its instincts. The key is to pay attention.

PHYSICAL SUPPORT FROM YOUR PARTNER

Doulas may be professionals who have a great deal of training and experience using certain physical techniques in the Natural Bag, but your partner can also implement simple and effective comfort measures during labor. Hand-holding and gentle touch and stroking are sometimes enough and just what is needed. Here are some other tools in your no-risk toolkit that your partner can perform:

- Using their hands for counter pressure, which can relieve back pain.
- Doing a "Double Hip Squeeze", also for back pain: While you are in a hands and knees position, or kneeling over the ball, your partner can kneel behind you, with the heels of their hands on your hips (the fleshy area at the top of your buttocks), fingers pointing toward each other, as their hands push in and together, in a slight upward direction.
- Massaging tense muscles – often in your neck, shoulders and back. Hand and foot massage is another stress reliever that may feel comforting in between contractions.
- Cuddling and kissing. You may only want this infrequently, or possibly not at all, but just know that this sort of intimate physical touch from your partner can increase the production of oxytocin, stimulating more effective contractions.

WATER

Water, as a tool in your Natural Bag, can be used in many ways. You can:

- Submerge yourself in a tub or birth pool.
- Have your partner pour water from a cup, slowly and rhythmically, over your back and/or belly, while you sit in a tub.

- Stand, lean against the wall or your partner, or sit on a bench or on the floor of the shower.
- Wet washcloths with cold or hot water (I love a Crockpot filled with water for this one!) and place on your body as desired. Cold usually feels good on your upper back, neck and forehead, and hot compresses are a significant pain reliever when placed low on your belly.

ENVIRONMENT

I touched on this earlier when discussing the physical setting in which you'll choose to give birth. No matter where that ends up being, you can set your environment up however you like, in order to be soothed and find strength, and remove tension triggers. Some ideas may include:

- Dim lighting
- Candles – for mood and/or scent
- Diffusers with essential oils
- Music – create playlists
- Surrounding yourself with the calm, encouraging, reassuring, kind, happy demeanor of your birth team

Your Medical Bag

Because there are always potential complications that can ensue with any of the tools in your Medical Bag, it's imperative that you make your choices wisely. If you try a certain position, sit on the birth ball, or get into the shower to ease pain and it doesn't work, you just move on to something else with no harm done. But when it comes to dipping your hand into the Medical Bag, more intricate decision-making strategies are needed. You must always be weighing your options, with the objective of benefit outweighing risk.

AMNIOTOMY

Amniotomy is the technical term for the artificial (intentional) rupture of the membranes, or breaking of the water, where an "amnihook" (a simple plastic device that looks like a long crochet hook) is used to snag and then tear the lower part of the amniotic sac, releasing the fluid. The desired goal with this procedure, if it is not being performed to facilitate another intervention, is to speed up labor. I know what you're thinking: "Yes, *please!*" Unfortunately, a routine amniotomy, performed for that particular outcome, is not evidence-based, meaning that it doesn't necessarily produce that result. As noted before, there's no fallout to experimenting with any of the tools in the Natural Bag, but when you reach into the Medical Bag and pull out the artificial rupturing of membranes, this can cause infection in the uterus, more intense contractions, more pain, and greater difficulty managing labor (which typically leads to more interventions). If your baby is not "engaged" in the pelvis, where their head is blocking the cervical opening, it is also possible for the umbilical cord to come down into, and sometimes out of, the vagina, once the sac is broken. This is called "cord prolapse", and it is a less common but more serious risk.

Here's one way of further understanding routine amniotomy. Imagine you're driving and running late for an appointment, so you press on the gas pedal, reasonably assuming that's how you'll get to your destination faster. In that moment your car accelerates, so your action feels validated. However, there are also police officers in unmarked cars behind the trees along your route, out of your view, and there's a traffic light a mile up the road. By deliberately speeding, you are risking being pulled over (adding more time to your trip and collecting an expensive traffic ticket), and/or getting into an accident. For incurring those potential threats and dangers, you might arrive home a couple of minutes sooner. But, in the end, you also have a 50/50 shot at getting stuck at the light and reaching your driveway at the same time you would have if you had stayed within the speed limit.

There are many scenarios that can take place during any particular labor, and any number of choices that could be made to resolve an unexpected occurrence – which is why knowing the specific risks and benefits of these tools is so vital. When you know what they are, you can consider them in the context of your uniquely unfolding labor.

So then, how can you choose this tool wisely? When does the benefit of "accelerating" prevail over the risk of "a ticket"? There are many scenarios that can take place during any particular labor, and any number of choices that could be made to resolve an unexpected occurrence – which is why knowing the specific risks and benefits of these tools is so vital. When you know what they are, you can consider them in the context of your uniquely unfolding labor. An amniotomy performed at the beginning of labor or when the cervix is still firm and mostly closed, is at a very different place on the pro/con scale than one executed later in labor, when the cervix is fully thinned out and open to, let's say, seven centimeters. But those are just a couple of distinctions. There are many other details to consider. Have other tools from the Natural Bag been implemented to augment a stalled, or very slowly progressing labor? Maybe your labor has continued to progress (your contractions are, unmistakably, longer, stronger, and closer together) and your baby has descended very far into the pelvis, but your cervix, although responsive to the work of your contractions, has plateaued at a juncture in which you'd expect it to be nearly ready for the pushing stage. This pretend, but realistic case, illustrates a time where the decision to access an amniotomy might make sense. It is reasonable to think that once the fluid from the bulging bag was released, and the baby's head put pressure on the cervix (already ripe and ready to fully open to 10 centimeters), your cervix would respond quickly. The fact that the membranes would not be ruptured for a prolonged period of time (as opposed to an amniotomy done early in labor) this risk of infection would be lower, and because the baby would have been engaged in the pelvis, the risk of cord prolapse would not exist. There will never be a guarantee that this is the right decision at the right time, which is why using your knowledge to make judgment calls is so important.

As we move on to look at other tools in the Medical Bag, and you imagine yourself making decisions during labor, it will be helpful for you to use this process of weighing pros and cons and determining if a particular choice would be warranted.

EPIDURAL

Epidural anesthesia is a regional anesthetic (numbing a large region of the body), but let's dispense with the formalities. Epidural anesthesia is the one tool in the Medical Bag that is praised and revered as if it was a literal godsend. The vast majority of birthing women can't possibly imagine going through labor without one. Nor can they fathom why anyone would. That makes perfect sense if, in line with all that has been cited, one is unaware that the Natural Bag exists, or that there can be significant risks associated with the options in the Medical Bag – even the option of an epidural, whose risks seem inconsequential when faced with pain you think cannot be managed in any other way.

Think about over-the-counter medication, or even prescription drugs which work to alleviate symptoms, most of the time. It would be unwise to take on the risks associated with them if those symptoms could be addressed in other effective, and harmless ways. I am not minimizing the practical miracle of eradicating acute pain, and I absolutely believe that medication has its place. However, there's simply no such thing as a free lunch.

The choice to pull an epidural from your Medical Bag should be just as calculated as any other decision you make. If we focus on the shared goal of avoiding an unnecessary C-section, choosing an epidural can either draw you away from or propel you toward that goal. Yes, you heard me correctly. Getting an epidural can actually save you from ending up with an unintended C-section. If the time you've been in labor, with no sleep and a reduced ability to manage your pain using the tools in your Natural Bag, begins to cause sheer exhaustion, if every last ounce of your energy is going toward survival, it is then prudent to respect the benefits of an epidural. This is certainly not comparable to the same epidural being chosen without first trying many, or even all of the tools in the Natural Bag, and when you still have the energy (although diminished) to work with your contractions in non-invasive ways. In that case, the risks will overtake the benefits.

An epidural will, in most cases, provide excellent pain relief. An epidural can also directly cause contractions to slow down and become inefficient, a decrease in blood pressure, itching, and fever, as well as lots of postpartum complications, such as long-term backaches and headaches, and numbness and tingling sensations. Indirectly, the low blood pressure sometimes experienced can affect the baby, your need to be immobile can further slow labor and inhibit the descent of your baby, and, the bladder catheter you receive, due to the inability to release urine, can lead to a bladder infection. A possible domino effect exists within each tool in the Medical Bag, which is a very good reason, in and of itself, to make your decisions with great thought and consideration, as opposed to the way many people will make their decisions – in ignorance, and with casual indifference. This is especially true when it comes to epidurals.

PITOCIN

Pitocin is the synthetic form of the hormone, oxytocin, which is produced in your body, and, for birth at least, is responsible for generating contractions.

There are many valid medical reasons for integrating pitocin as a means to augment or induce labor. In these isolated instances, you could expect your doctor or midwife to thoroughly review their assessments and recommendations, and, of course, you could also ask many questions and avail yourself of the medical literature to feel comfortable with your final decision.

In the vast majority of situations, a birthing woman's body will produce enough oxytocin to generate effective contractions from early labor through the delivery of the placenta. During times in which contractions are not leading to progress, pitocin, as a tool in your Medical Bag, can be used to augment your labor. The disadvantages of choosing pitocin to intensify existing contractions and speed up labor are much the same as some of the disadvantages of choosing an Amniotomy to produce an equivalent outcome. Pitocin can cause abnormally strong contractions that may also come very close together. With the sudden onset of increased pain and shorter breaks, labor becomes more difficult to manage, which may require a cascade of additional interventions. Your baby may not "like" the effects of pitocin either. Intense contractions that last longer than normal can cause an unnatural reduction in oxygen. Some fetuses will show signs of distress if these reactions occur.

There are many tools in the Natural Bag that can be used to augment a stalled labor. If you assess your own situation and conclude that the benefits of using pitocin would outweigh the risks, you may end up choosing this tool for that purpose. It is reassuring to know that you and your baby will be monitored, and that the level of pitocin, delivered through an IV, can be lowered or shut off, if its effects are detrimental to either of you. This is yet another reason why it's necessary for you to know what is in the Natural Bag, even if you don't plan on having a natural birth. Although it is much wiser to use the Medical Bag as a backup, if you choose it as your primary toolkit and you then lose an opportunity to use an item, like pitocin, for instance, you either substitute it with natural tools, or you head for the operating room.

Pitocin can also be chosen alone or as part of a set of tools to induce labor, before you start having contractions. An important part of the decision-making process should be to consider the following: If your cervix is somewhat soft, open, and in position (anterior), pitocin can get labor going by stimulating contractions. If your cervix is still thick, closed, and facing backward (posterior), pitocin will cause contractions, but they are less likely to be productive.

There are certain people, under certain circumstances, who choose to be induced, even in situations where evidence would not support the decision. Being "done" with a pregnancy or wanting to ensure that one particular doctor from the practice you're using will be at your birth, are two examples of this. As always, there is no judgment on my part. You've probably started to realize just how personal everything about birth is, or at least should be. My view is that no matter how much evidence exists, pointing toward the "best way", there are unique factors that cannot be subjected to rigorous research, but are, still, valid parts of what constitutes an ultimate birth experience. As long as you are aware of the evidence and you combine it with all of the other emotional, physical, relational and environmental pieces, you will make the best decisions for yourself.

Years ago, one of my students approached me after class quite upset. She had lost her mother when she was young and was very close with her father. She lived in New York and her dad lived in Florida. He had a job in which he could only take off a specified amount of time and he requested this time around his daughter's due date, hoping he would be able to arrive shortly before she gave birth, and then spend some time with her and his new grandchild before returning home. This would also serve as a significant source of emotional support for her. As her pregnancy advanced, she began to feel concerned with the prospect of going into labor later than her due date. This would mean that her father would spend most of his time with her before the baby was born, or that he might miss the birth entirely.

The reason for her distress was that she now understood the risks of induction, especially as there was no medical need to choose this path, and she was conflicted over what to do. Being educated comes with responsibilities that many will resist, but those who recognize the tremendous associated benefits that accompany knowledge, will be rewarded many times over for the mental effort it takes to make these difficult decisions. And that's just what she had set herself up for. She was positioned to construct a comprehensive list of pros and cons that included both physical and emotional aspects. On one hand, she didn't want to inflate her risk of a difficult labor and the increased outcome of a C-section, and on the other hand, she knew she would be devastated if her experience did not involve her dad, in the way she had hoped. She thought about it. She worked through it extensively, with me, with family and friends, and on her own. She decided to request a vaginal exam at 38 weeks, a few days before her father's arrival, to see what, if anything, was happening with her cervix. Once she found out that her body had done enough in advance of labor to create favorable conditions for success (her cervix had softened, moved forward and opened a bit), she decided to schedule an induction. There were still potential risks that someone else might not have taken, and there were no guarantees that the induction would go smoothly. However, the beauty of this story is twofold. One, she fully understood the importance of putting her personal needs and values into the equation. Two, she knew how to choose and use a medical tool in a way that fit in with her unique circumstances.

The induction was ultimately successful. She had a vaginal birth, her father was there, and he was able to stay for almost two weeks after her baby girl was born. Regardless of how this played out, she would have had no regrets, for she was equipped with the knowledge she needed to choose her own path, having taken everything into consideration, especially what she personally valued most.

CHOOSING BETWEEN BAGS

You are an active participant in your birth, able to make decisions and use resources that will coincide with what will be helpful *in the moment* (the only time you can make these choices), and you don't have to pick sides. It is not necessary to have both feet in the "all natural" camp or the "all medical intervention" camp.

In case you're still stuck on the impressive nature of medical techniques and drugs for pain relief, I need you to extend some trust. The items in the Natural Bag work, so please don't disregard them. The best advice I can give you is to use those natural tools *first*, not necessarily *only*. If you're planning to give birth in a hospital, you will eventually have access to all of the tools in the Medical Bag, but you will probably be laboring at home for a while, during which time that bag will remain sealed. So, regardless of your eventual intentions, knowing how to use the contents of the Natural Bag is essential.

When faced with a fork in the road of your plan or idea of how your birth will progress; when Mother Nature decides to exert her authority, you need not be paralyzed and unable to pivot. You will know of and be able to use the tools to work with your labor in that moment.

Those of you who are not necessarily interested in a natural birth but would still like to avoid routine interventions and the potential snowball effects of those interventions (leading to more interventions you didn't purposely choose), have a whole toolkit to start with. If a natural birth is your goal, you still get to walk into your labor with the Medical Bag. No one is taking it away from you. It's your choice if and when to use one or all of the tools within.

Plus, you do not have to soldier through your pain just because it's your choice not to have an epidural. There are so many non-invasive comfort measures you can choose from.

DO WHAT FEELS RIGHT

I've concentrated, to a great extent, on the physical aspects of how to apply your toolkits in labor. Equal in significance is how implementing this will affect the mental and emotional side of giving birth. The medical management of labor, in which your care providers check off a predetermined list of procedures to expedite the process, renders your role in your own birth virtually worthless. They call all the shots and make all the decisions. Sadly, this has become acceptable, for fear that if we don't just do as we're told and follow a script, we and our babies will be in danger; or because of the lack of interest in the effort that must be put into taking responsibility for ourselves. Maybe it's a combination of both. Please don't be lazy. And please quit perpetuating the concept of "doctor as savior". This keeps you small and vulnerable and unable to take control of your own experience. If you open your mind and your brain to learning about the toolkits you possess; if you discover them, blow off the dust, and explore each of their various features, you will not have to rely on someone else to tell you how to best manage your unique

If you open your mind and your brain to learning about the toolkits you possess; if you discover them, blow off the dust, and explore each of their various features, you will not have to rely on someone else to tell you how to best manage your unique labor – your pain and your progress.

labor – *your* pain and *your* progress. This will, without a doubt, give you a tremendous sense of control and confidence.

Moreover, I urge you not to get caught up in some man-made version of "dignity" at the expense of working with your body in a primal way - a way that will make your labor easier and facilitate progress. As a doula, I had an interesting and sort of funny situation occur a while back. Upon arriving at the hospital, my client affirmed she wanted a wheelchair when asked, as she was in very active labor and her contractions were intense and coming frequently. The volunteer who showed up with the wheelchair, and who would escort us to the labor and delivery area of the hospital, was a cheerful, gentle, older woman. Into the elevator we all went, followed by a couple of other people. Within seconds, a contraction began, and out of the wheelchair, down on all fours, this amazing laboring mom went! While she began to rock and moan, the poor, elderly volunteer became wide-eyed and flustered. "Miss, Miss, you need to get back in the wheelchair," she gasped. "The floor is dirty and you're going to get hurt!" So sweet. So well-meaning. But so misguided.

See birth for what it is – a completely normal, physiological event in your life; an event that should be overseen and monitored to circumvent occasional anomalies and barriers, but one that is respected for its proficiency. See yourself as the leader, not the follower, of this magnificent and paramount voyage. Learn how to use the resources you can access, and then choose them as you see fit. Collaborate with your team, expecting that they may make suggestions, offer guidance and recommend certain tools, and that you always, ultimately, get to decide for yourself.

WHAT NOW?

○ Learn - dive into your options, know the pros and cons, the benefits and risks of each tool in your Natural and Medical Bags.

○ Consider ways you might make decisions during your labor, imagining yourself using these tools.

○ Get prepared - gather up some of the resources from your Natural Bag that you might want to have on hand, such as:
  • Birth Ball
  • Washcloths
  • Crockpot
  • Diffuser and essential oils
  • Birthing tub/pool
  • Candles
  • Music playlist(s)
  • Massage tools
  • Drinks and Snacks

○ Partner – learn about all support techniques, and then practice physical ones, such as the Double Hip Squeeze.

Thoughts and Actions

_____

_____

_____

_____

_____

_____

_____

_____

_____

_____

_____

_____

_____

_____

Chapter 6

OF COURSE YOU SHOULD PLAN YOUR BIRTH

"Plans are nothing; planning is everything."
- DWIGHT D. EISENHOWER

I got engaged fourteen months before my wedding day. In that span of time, I spent hundreds of hours getting ready for, what would be, a five-hour celebration. Visiting catering facilities, bridal shops and florists, choosing a photographer, a band and the music we would want them to play, picking out, and then preparing and mailing the invitations, deciding who would be our bridesmaids and groomsmen and what they would wear, organizing a registry, selecting the menu. From large arrangements to small details, the planning seemed endless.

Even if you have never planned a wedding, at some point in your life you will have attended some function that was the culmination of a great deal of planning. Whether lavish parties or backyard celebrations, weddings usually require a good deal of preparation for an event that will be over in what seems like a blink of an eye. Where is the sense in that? Why do we do it?

The answer lies in the value we place on that moment in time and our perception of the worth of a desired outcome. In planning, we focus on what we care about and assemble that which we have control over, all the while taking a subconscious leap of faith, knowing our efforts will get us as close as possible to a sought-after goal, but will, undoubtedly, fall short of perfection.

The planning of a wedding involves researching and questioning. As choices arise, the process of planning reveals what is most personally valuable - where there's a will to compromise and where there is not. We are given this amazing opportunity to learn how to productively communicate and negotiate, how to take control and remain flexible at the same time.

We don't assume that planning is a waste of time simply because there are no guarantees. We don't feel foolish when we devote great heaps of energy to a specific outcome, knowing the possibility that the outcome will not be realized. In hindsight, it is always the planned experience that gives way to a reflection of pride and satisfaction. Only the affairs we leave to chance embody the probability of regret.

Only the affairs we leave to chance embody the probability of regret.

You may have been under the assumption that you cannot

110

plan your birth in the same way that one would plan a wedding. Why? Because you're not intelligent enough to research? Because there are no choices?

On the other hand, you may know you *could* plan your birth, but you resist doing so because you feel there is only one safe way, making your possible desires selfish and, perhaps, dangerous. Or, if you plan, it will raise your hopes and you don't want to be disappointed. Or you're just simply too intimidated to relay your preferences to your doctor.

The stakes are high, my friend. Dare I say that planning a birth trumps planning a wedding many times over? Apathy, fear, and assumptions have no place in birth.

You are most certainly intelligent enough to research, to understand and to make sense of the many choices you have. You've now begun to see how the common perceptions of the path toward a safe birth are often unsound and untrue. To back away from planning your birth because you're afraid of disappointment is to remove every profound benefit planning embodies, and to position yourself perfectly for misgiving.

If you fail to communicate what this birth means to you and your expectations for it, then the experience, in all ways, will be navigated by someone else – someone with their own personal beliefs about birth, and their own agendas, having nothing to do with yours.

Concealing your wishes when you're giving birth in a hospital – which is not just an establishment to treat illness and address medical events, but an institution with business practices, and protocols to foster the bottom line and generate income – will allow these business practices and protocols to dictate how your birth is manifested. This is not to detract from the remarkable work that takes place in hospitals all day, every day. I don't mean to devalue the important and honorable work of medical professionals or administrators. The hospital must be run as a business in order to exist in its intended capacity, with the bulk of that business coming from "customers" requiring treatment, procedures, remedies and surgeries. Most birthing people, comprised of low-risk women encountering a normal, physiological process, may require the safeguards this business can offer, but even so, not all to the same extent. A mechanic who specializes in engine-rebuilds, and has an automated system for efficiency and productivity, can still change your oil and rotate your tires, but if you drop off your car without communicating that you just want your oil changed and your tires rotated, be prepared to have your engine rebuilt.

Your care providers are not mind readers, and their practices, like hospitals, are also businesses. There are systems in place for their personal benefit, for the benefit of their organization, and for those they serve. They have lots and lots of patients. They may listen if you speak. They may take the time to discuss your preferences if you convey them. They may respect your wishes if you make them known. Even when engaging with the most supportive doctors and midwives, they will not remember what you desire unless you take the steps to be remembered. Open up the lines of communication between you and your birth team, including and especially your medical caregivers. Help them to understand your values around birth and what is important to you. This gives them the opportunity to support you as an individual. It also affords you and your partner the chance to "feel out" your practitioner's view of, and mindset around birth. This will ensure that you are on the same page, or it will elicit further discussion, or it will raise a red flag for the possible need to make changes to your birth team.

Dive into the planning of your birth and you will surely get closer to your dreams, all the while enriching the entire experience. Remove the anxiety around pain and the fear of imagined complications, and you're left with feelings of pure happiness and excitement around having your baby. As with every momentous celebration, every joyful milestone, much of the fun and exhilaration is in the planning. This is an amazing opportunity to forge a deeper bond with your partner. Determining your shared values and developing your wish list together will help you to become aligned and establish the space in which to work through personal ideas and emotions. You will be rewarded with a heightened sense of confidence, as planning your birth brings awareness to how much you've learned, not only about labor and birth, but about yourself. Sensing the gravity of your reasonable requests and having your expectations heard and respected will motivate you to continue communicating with tenacity, not just for this birth, but for future births and in all of life's journeys.

A REALITY CHECK

Unfortunately, birth plans have a tarnished reputation. Based on the common rhetoric known to birth workers, it seems that the disdain for birth plans originated with prickly relationships between demanding clients who were expecting guarantees, and ego-driven providers who were not interested in rights and requests outside of their standard practices, regardless of how reasonable those requests might have been. And so, the birth plan and those who wrote birth plans were vilified. But that has nothing to do with you as a consumer of the ultimate birth experience, because you understand how off-the-charts crazy it would be to show up to the most important moment of your life without a plan. You, who spent hours researching and sorting through the differences between UPPAbaby and Bugaboo strollers. You know how essential it is to establish some kind of plan for your birth.

So, even though I'm going to lay out the behind-the-scenes reality that often corrupts the stellar intentions of a birth plan, please don't back down. Don't allow this to cause more intimidation. Do not shrink away from planning your birth.

This may seem difficult to believe, but behind women's backs, jokes are often made about those who come to the hospital with a birth plan. Nurses sometimes make off-hand comments about how the woman with the birth plan is destined for a C-section, even mocking these women to their faces. This is not okay. If anyone is making fun of your birth plan, they are making fun of you. Keep that in mind when your vulnerable self begins to question whether or not you're actually foolish for thinking you have a right to ask for what you want. The fact that some women don't have any preferences or care all that much about their birth experiences, does not make it wrong or inappropriate for you, especially when those preferences are steeped in thoughtful consideration and education.

It is downright disgusting that you would ever be made to feel ridiculous for presenting your plan, not to mention expecting support of that plan. Imagine engaging with a travel agent to put together the details for an upcoming trip. Think of yourself sitting down with her to discuss your list. Let's say there are four people in your family – you, your husband, your three-year-old son and your infant daughter. Your husband has back issues and your son can't eat gluten. You want to go someplace warm, with activities suitable for your little boy, and accommodations on one level so your husband doesn't have to carry bags or the kids up and down stairs. You're not really a beach person, so you want someplace with a pool. And so on. You wouldn't arbitrarily get on a plane to somewhere and hope for the best when you land. Can the travel agent guarantee good weather? Is it her fault if the resort changed its menu the day before you arrived, and they no longer have gluten-free options? Of course not. Would it be reasonable for you to expect this travel agent to listen, to guide you, to work with you, and to support your choices? Absolutely. How would you feel if she said, "Anything can happen, so stop stressing over every detail, and leave everything to me. You *think* you want a pool. Everyone says that, but once they get there, they realize they'd rather have the beach."

If you're thinking, "Well, birth is totally different than a vacation", it is either because you're still of the mindset that you can't state your wishes for any medical event (which birth generally isn't, or shouldn't be, most of the time) or because you are still equating a birth plan with your fantasy about how your experience will evolve.

Birth is usually a low-risk physiological event, and so you have as many choices and as much of a right to make those choices as you do when planning a vacation. Even when it's not a low-risk situation, you still have choices. You would just need to work within more narrow guidelines to create your plan, but you are, nevertheless, entitled to the options available to you. Only in very rare situations, where there is an emergency medical crisis, would you, potentially, have to surrender nearly all of your birth plan, and even then, there are choices that would still be attainable. You could conceivably salvage your desire to have doula support, or save your placenta for encapsulation, or keep your request for 24-hour rooming in, as a few examples.

The idea that we have made it acceptable to snicker at a person's desire to experience something that is so personal, meaningful, and transformational, is appalling. It's as if those doling out the eye-rolling believe that they are the keepers of some hidden secret, some inside joke, because they've seen lots and lots of women in labor changing their minds about not having an epidural. That does not, in any way, mean that it's idiotic to plan for and work toward a birth without medication. Gosh, we have all been judged in situations that were not as soul-baring as giving birth, and we know how demeaning and shameful it feels to be condemned and ridiculed for our goals, especially when, for one reason or another, those goals don't materialize. So, are we to simply shuffle into the hospital with our heads down and our mouths shut, like good little patients?

Even those who don't necessarily have a formal birth plan but question routine practices and hesitate to submit to popular choices without some contemplation, are often met with condescension. One of my colleagues, now a seasoned birth professional, was not fully informed prior to having her first baby, but had a deep intuition around birth and birth practices. She recounts, "I was mocked by the nursing staff when I said, well I don't know how I feel yet… maybe I would like an epidural… can you tell me before it's too late? 'Aw honey, they all say that', the nurse said to me. 'You're cute. Yeah, I'll go tell the anesthesiologist to get ready now.'"

There are actually hashtags ridiculing birth plans, including #birthplansareajoke and #birthplanssuck. I had to check out the corresponding posts to see where these were coming from. Apparently, those who don't believe in birth plans, including some wonderful birth workers, view the term "plan" as a set of strict ideas and guidelines that, already stressed-out, pregnant mamas are setting their sights on with rigid expectations. They seem to think that the definition of a birth plan is what I would define as a birth fantasy – how you might hope your birth will go in your imagination - which I still think is perfectly appropriate! I just want you to make the distinction between the two.

When I was planning my home birth, I intended on having my husband make a fire in the fireplace at some point. I was due in January, and I envisioned myself laboring by the cozy fireplace, watching, and being soothed by the flames. But, on that particular day, it was over 60 degrees in New York, and although my husband still asked, there would have been nothing comforting about being extremely hot while dealing with contractions, so that part of the plan went by the wayside.

Fantasies are healthy and fun, but not so much if you consider them your fixed plan. Know the difference between daydreaming and navigating the system in order to increase the probability of getting what you want.

I would agree that you can't plan when or how you're going to go into labor, or exactly how this labor will come to pass, but that is not the intention of a birth plan. Do you not plan your wedding, knowing the likelihood that certain things may go off course? Do you abandon your plan for a wedding on the beach because you have no control over whether or not it rains that day? If it does indeed rain, do you think, "What a waste all that planning was?" Some people take exception to the word "plan", feeling it's more appropriate to refer to a list of "preferences". I say it's all semantics, and I'm not sure why the term represents such a terrifying commitment.

Your birth plan is never written in stone, since planning necessarily requires flexibility. The intention is not for you to compromise in order to appease your doctor. It's for you, so that you can walk into your birth with a mixture of strength in your convictions and realistic expectations. My hope is that you will gain the knowledge and embrace the wisdom you need to change gears when you recognize that doing so will serve you in the long run. If you need to shift and relinquish an anticipated objective, you will understandably be disappointed, but I pray you'll be able to focus on the strength and acumen it takes to alter your path, as opposed to the unreasonable feelings of failure. I long for you to have total support, encouragement and praise from each person on your birth team, who respects and believes in your choices, and lifts you up as you courageously make difficult, unexpected decisions you might not have wanted to make.

On many occasions I've had the honor of working with women attempting to heal from previous birth traumas. Although they may not have been entirely scarred from their first births, they often came away from those experiences knowing it could have been better, more empowering, and less distressing. Many times, there is this vague sense that something just wasn't "right" – that if they had known what their choices were and how to advocate for those choices, they would have felt better about themselves in one way or another, or they would have had a better physical outcome. Almost always, these stories involve other individuals taking the choices out of their hands (choices they may not have even known they had) and controlling their experience. When they learn of those choices, after the fact, and how to implement them, they have a deep feeling of loss and regret. My stance here, as it is in virtually every aspect of birth, is that it's all a lesson for the future. You can't go backwards, but once you recognize that there are different approaches you could take for your next birth, once you are introduced to new concepts and opportunities, you could very well have a cathartic and restorative experience which prompts you to take back and strengthen your power.

A story that exemplifies this involves a woman I taught and supported through the labor and birth of her second baby. She wanted to have a natural birth the first time and ended up with both an epidural and pitocin. The repercussions were not catastrophic, but she harbored a feeling of loss – not only a loss of her goals and her ability to see her birth plan carried out – but an overall loss of control and confidence. Without a specific understanding of how she could have managed her labor differently, she was unable to put her finger on what changes she needed to make the second time around. We met prior to this second pregnancy. Over the course of some informal discussions around birth, her eyes would light up as she was beginning to make connections between what had happened, why she was having these feelings, and what she could change in the future. Within a few months she was pregnant and putting her resolve into practice. She sought out a practitioner who would offer informed choices and individualized care. She surrounded herself with other like-minded birth professionals who would add to her knowledge base while boosting her confidence and protecting her vision. I had the privilege of providing education, resources, and coaching to her and her husband as the pregnancy continued, and then the humbling honor of attending her birth as their doula. She walked into this birth with the insight and courage to see her plan through. However, as we've been discussing, there is no amount of preparation that can guarantee any experience in life, birth or otherwise, progressing without a hitch.

Fast forward to the day she went into labor: her contractions were unusually strong and painful from the start. Although she used many tools from the Natural Bag, and her mental will to work with her body was unwavering, the sheer amount of time she was dealing with atypical contractions was wearing her down. In addition, she had a low-lying placenta, which was being watched closely and could have caused complications leading to a C-section. Her options were presented to her, and then left entirely to her discretion. Ultimately, she chose an epidural (to alleviate pain and stress with the intention of facilitating progress, and in case she ended up needing a C-section emergently). Because her contractions became somewhat ineffective, she also chose a measured dose of pitocin.

Labor progressed and she had a beautiful, vaginal birth. Even so, she cried as she surrendered to the two interventions she had had in her first birth, and then, for a time after her precious baby was born. Her initial perception was that of defeat, but that changed as soon as she could internalize how very different the circumstances were: knowledge versus ignorance, advocacy versus resignation, informed decisions versus passive management, being in control versus being powerless. Once the clarity set in, once she was able to debrief and process the entire experience, she recognized how thoroughly dissimilar her two births were, even with the same procedures she so much wanted to avoid the second time. She realized that she had *proactively* pulled those procedures from the Medical Bag, using a calculated benefit/risk decision-making process, as opposed to accepting them just because her midwife told her to. The plan, if simply defined by the list of preferences, was nothing. It had very little to do with achieving the ultimate birth experience. The planning, on the other hand - the massive amount of attitude change, thought, time and effort - would open up her whole world and transform her in ways she never expected.

> *The plan, if simply defined by the list of preferences, was nothing. It had very little to do with achieving the ultimate birth experience. The planning, on the other hand - the massive amount of attitude change, thought, time and effort - would open up her whole world and transform her in ways she never expected.*

HOW TO WRITE AND DISCUSS A BIRTH PLAN

The first thing you must do when writing a birth plan, or just figuring out what you want and what you don't want, is to tap into your values. Decide what is most important to you. Decide what is firm, where you will not make concessions, barring any need to address a medical concern, in which plan B would be evidence-based, justifying the surrendering of your ideals. You must also have some education about birth, including common interventions during labor. Without thorough knowledge a birth plan is just a wish list. You can't expect to be able to make decisions in the moment when the circumstances change. It's difficult, if not impossible, to confidently advocate for what you want when you're unfamiliar with the evidence. Without knowing your options and the pros, cons, and alternatives associated with these options, you'll be unable to implement the steps toward your goals.

Once you have the confidence to ask for what you want, there are some guidelines you might find helpful.

Have an understanding of the position your doctor or midwife is in, which does not mean that you back down. This sense of empathy will be useful in your communication skills. Remember, the goal is not just to write a plan, or get through the appointment where you discuss your plan. It's either to – hopefully, fingers-crossed – secure full, genuine support, with or without some compromise, or to recognize that you will not be supported, which could prompt the need for a change in provider.

Aim for a combination of protecting your plan and your rights, with an appropriate dose of flexibility. Demanding and expecting guarantees is not only unreasonable, but it will create a divide between you and the person from whom you're trying to gain consideration, agreement, and support.

As an example, if after achieving a full understanding of the evidence around Electronic Fetal Monitoring, you conclude that the best and safest approach for you and your baby is to have intermittent monitoring, with the option to freely move around and change positions, you might approach the conversation like this:

> *Once I arrive at the hospital and I have the monitor on just long enough to determine that the baby is doing well, I would like to have intermittent monitoring and the freedom to move around and change positions. I understand that if I choose an epidural, I will need to have the monitor on continuously. If there is an*

unforeseen medical situation in which continuous monitoring would be beneficial, I would like this recommendation to be discussed with me and my partner, and the risks, benefits, and alternatives to be shared beforehand.

The response you're hoping for is:

Based on the evidence around fetal monitoring, and the fact that your pregnancy is low-risk, I don't want you to be strapped to that monitor your entire labor! We will get a tracing when you get to the hospital, and then we'll encourage you to do whatever feels best and brings you the most comfort. Our protocol is to monitor the baby intermittently, and I will step in only if there's a medical need. Not only then, but always, I will seek to keep you in control and make sure I provide what you need to make informed choices.

It is critical, when having these discussions around your plan and preferences, to be able to distinguish between being supported and tolerated; to differentiate between having your wishes respected and being placated. I've been reminding you that you are a consumer, and although the service you are purchasing is unlike any other, make no mistake – there is still marketing involved in this transaction. The most likely scenario is that the "seller" has a mix of your best interests in mind, as well as their own. Depending on their general view of birth, how they perceive the definition of a successful "deal", and their negotiating strategies:

o   You may be intimidated into feeling you must trust them as the expert if you want a safe outcome - based on their goal to practice in the easiest, most efficient manner, without challenge of any kind, and/or to be protected from a lawsuit; or,

○ You may be appeased and temporarily satisfied with an agreement that has a fragile backbone – based on the underlying conviction that birth is inherently dangerous, and the notion that what you're asking for is reasonable on paper but will probably go out the window once the serious business of labor begins; or,

○ You may be respected and fully supported without judgment – based on this person's genuine belief that they are in a partnership with their patients, that it is the birthing person who should remain in command, and because they possess a view of birth as sacred and deserving of honor.

The best advice I can offer is to ask very specific "devil's advocate" type of questions, and to use your intuition. What I want for you, and what I would think you want for yourself, is to know that you and your baby and your birth experience are nurtured in a way that never has you second-guessing your team's sincerity or their commitment to individualized, evidence-based, unbiased care.

On a purely strategic level of presenting your birth plan, you want to make sure you have the time to do so and you have your provider's undivided attention. That may seem difficult if you're used to the standard practice of 10-minute prenatal appointments. Here is all you need to do: call the office and ask for extra time in an upcoming appointment. Let them know you have some things to discuss which you'd like to do after your exam (ideally in an office, as opposed to in the room where you're sitting on an exam table and your partner is squeezed into a corner). Do not, in any way, feel uneasy or intimidated about asking for this! It's probable that they don't get this request very often, because the majority of expectant people are still assuming that there's nothing to talk about. Unlike you, they are not investigating their options, advocating for their preferences, or contemplating their birth experience at all, and therefore, don't have a reason to schedule longer appointments. That's ok. You're done toeing the line and basing your actions on what everyone else is doing or not doing. This is a reasonable and appropriate consumer-to-provider appeal. Ask. It could very well be the start of a much-needed flexing of your communication and advocacy muscles.

Do not be surprised if you get some pushback. Your doctor or midwife may not agree with all of your preferences. It's appropriate, and important, to keep an open mind and hear them out. What's not appropriate is being made to feel as if you are not capable of having a reasonable, intelligent, informed discussion about the topics you want to review because you are not an obstetrician or midwife. You are certainly able to research and learn (which I highly encourage you to do before opening up the lines of communication) whether or not you have a medical degree. In the introduction to *Obstetric Myths Versus Research Realities*, author Henci Goer relays this story to explain her capacity and justification in writing a book that deals, to a large extent, in medical matters surrounding pregnancy, labor, and birth:

> *What's not appropriate is being made to feel as if you are not capable of having a reasonable, intelligent, informed discussion about the topics you want to review because you are not an obstetrician or midwife.*

"Penny Simkin, well-known educator, writer, speaker, and editor, was called on the carpet by an anesthesiologist, irate that she had written a handout listing the potential trade-offs of epidural anesthesia when she was not a doctor (although he did not dispute her accuracy.) 'What are your credentials?' he demanded. 'I can read,' was her reply. So can I. For that matter, you can too."

So, by all means, try not to put your guard up, but be bold in your convictions when your requests are meaningful to you, and especially when they are supported by evidence.

In the end, it's not about whether you have a natural birth or a medicated birth, a vaginal birth or a C-section. Your plan is a plan, not a contract. The expectation is that circumstances will not occur precisely as you thought or laid out, but the *planning* is key. The more informed you are, the more you communicate with your caregivers *before* labor begins, the more you discuss and agree upon your ideals with your partner, the more prepared your birth team is, the higher the chance of reaching the ultimate goal of a safe and satisfying birth.

WHAT NOW?

○ Get informed. (I know, I sound like a broken record).

○ Communicate with your partner. Decide what is most important to you, where you might be willing to compromise and where you're not.

○ Feel free to find a template for a birth plan online, but it's not necessary. Write notes to reference when you verbally communicate and then add more details if you wish to submit a written copy.

○ Review this chapter for communication tips.

Thoughts and Actions

_____

_____

_____

_____

_____

_____

_____

_____

_____

_____

_____

Chapter 7

YOUR RIGHTS REDUCE YOUR RISK

"Birth should not be a time in a woman's life when she has to fight for anything."

— CARLA HARTLEY

Most of you know you have basic human rights, constitutional rights, and rights to equality. You may have even needed to defend those rights at one point, or at many points in your life. What you may not know is that your rights extend to birth, not only from a moral perspective, but a legal one as well.

If evidence-based care was actually practiced the majority of the time, you might be able to put less thought into this, but that is not the case. Standard, routine care, especially in hospital births (which constitute over 98% of all births) is at odds with evidence-based care. Most care is made up of practices that have perpetuated merely because of tradition and underlying agendas. These practices are not supported by science.

I know this is not what you want to hear. Subconsciously, no one, as a consumer of medical care, wants to think that anything will ever go wrong. When having a baby, you don't ever want to consider the alternatives to a smooth birth experience and a healthy outcome. So, the idea that those caring for you might be fallible human beings, who are not all-knowing and all-powerful, is unacceptable, and the belief that you will be guaranteed the result you expect if you put your trust in your doctor, is comforting. Herein lies the reason why many, if not most expecting women and their partners will never even think about their rights, much less research what those rights are, and advocate for their adherence.

The fact is, our legal rights in the birth arena are largely unclear to both expectant parents and providers, and they are frequently ignored. Violations of the legal and human rights practice of informed consent occur more often than informed consent is actually enforced. Here is an example: a doctor checks the birthing woman's cervix and says, "If there's no progress in an hour I'll break your water." No discussion of benefits, risks, or alternatives – just a proclamation of the doctor's plan.

Not that it makes it justifiable, but most care providers don't realize they are violating informed consent. This is how they were trained. Labor and delivery nurses, for instance, learn the routines that have to be performed when a patient arrives at the hospital. They are generally not instructed to discuss pros and cons and ask the patient for their consent. Rather, they must go through the list as efficiently as possible. Instead of discussing the benefits, risks, and alternatives of the IV, the nurse will typically announce that one is being given. Even the patient gown, although not a medical procedure, is an example of a practice for which no options are considered or offered. You rarely hear, "Would you like to put on this gown or wear something you've brought from home?"

When we talk about informed consent, we're really talking about informed consent and refusal. The relevance of informed consent comes from your right to say "no", with or without justification. You may very well agree with or be willing to compromise on a suggested medical procedure or intervention after a discussion in which you feel fully informed. *You don't have to refuse a* You may agree that an IV is a *recommendation in order to* good idea for hydration, and *uphold your rights. Likewise,* something you want, if you've *it does not make you* been unable to keep liquids *"difficult" or "rebellious" if* down and the benefits and *you decide to decline.* risks are explained to you. You don't have to refuse a recommendation in order to uphold your rights. Likewise, it does not make you "difficult" or "rebellious" if you decide to decline.

Unfortunately, when medical procedures are discussed, there is little to no provision of information about risks and potential benefits, so the delivery of the message comes off as a certainty or a mandate, not a suggestion. You may feel intimidated by an overconfident attitude, and you may not have any information going into that discussion. If so, you will automatically make the assumption that this procedure or intervention has no risks, that there are no choices, and that the benefits to your baby are absolute and undeniable. In this common occurrence the thought process is typically: "Why would I say "no" when this can benefit me and my baby?" Without preparatory information in the form of independent learning, and with the rampant exclusion of informed consent, it's not possible to have any other viewpoint. It's not possible to recognize that this may, in truth, *not* necessarily help you or your baby, and *could* sabotage those efforts, and even cause harm.

It's also important to note that you don't forfeit your rights when you walk through the hospital doors, and you don't forfeit your rights when you sign consent forms.

Don't confuse the consent form with informed consent. Remember, informed consent involves an in-the-moment discussion of pros, cons, alternatives, and the pros and cons of the alternatives. Nowhere in a consent form is this level of detail provided. Rather, it is written as a simple assertion of your acceptance. It is not legally binding. Furthermore, contrary to what some believe to be true, and what is perpetuated as truth, just because you sign a consent form, it does not take the place of informed consent, and it does not withdraw or supersede your rights. Consent forms are utilized for the protection of hospitals and care providers, rather than to preserve your rights. You can change your mind at any time during your labor. Unless you are unconscious and harm is imminent without treatment, you have the same right of refusal that you would have in any other healthcare situation, and any other life situation. "No" means "no", whether you have signed a form or not.

Many years ago, my friend was having her second baby. Her labor was progressing quickly. When she got to the hospital she was met by a resident and agreed to a vaginal exam to check her dilation.

While undergoing this exam, he chose to rupture her amniotic sac without mentioning his intentions or alerting her in advance. Not only was there no discussion initiated by this doctor, and no informed consent given by my friend, constituting a complete violation of her rights, but I want to further emphasize that this procedure was one involving physical contact with her genitals - penetration of her vagina - as do many of the procedures that are often part of pregnancy, labor, and birth. However unpleasant you may find a vaginal exam, it may feel acceptable to acquiesce to a highly personal medical examination when it benefits and safeguards your health and the well-being of your baby. But especially when it is an optional, arbitrary *choice*, with no evidence-based justification, to have anyone, in the healthcare arena or otherwise, do anything on, in, or remotely close to your vagina, I would hope you'd insist on consent – informed or not. For without that consent, let's be sure to call it what it is. Assault.

It's possible that I've riled you up a bit. But am I telling you all this to incite rage? To make you paranoid and militant? Certainly not. I encourage you to come from a place of trust, as I expect that you'll assemble your birth team and choose your place of birth after a great deal of vetting, and that you will have established that trust, wherever you can, in advance. Protecting and defending your rights is not only an action you take when those rights are being threatened. It's something you do just by expecting honesty and full disclosure. I often think that care providers and hospital administrators would be eager to guarantee the practice of informed consent, and that it would be upheld without exception. In my mind, it would alleviate the unreasonable responsibility that is often placed on medical professionals and hospitals. But the vicious cycle of consumers of healthcare demanding perfect outcomes, and medical providers believing that they can and should accommodate that absurd expectation, keeps the system where it is. The stage was set a long time ago, and it goes both ways. By shrugging off the options to become knowledgeable, to plan, and to advocate, birthing people have, generally, abandoned personal accountability for their own experiences. Doctors, then, respond by taking over, which threatens the rights of their patients. In the other direction, doctors have initiated this idea that they know what's right and best for all, and there's no need to educate and inform. Birthing people, consequently, don't think to, or are afraid of questioning and seeking alternatives, which, in practice, deprives them of their rights altogether.

When rights are not respected, outcomes are worse – not just physical outcomes, but mental and emotional outcomes as well. The fallout can be extreme if you are coerced, disrespected, condemned, belittled, victimized, bullied, ignored, or punished for speaking up or refusing to follow standard protocol. The prevalence of social injustice is high with certain social and ethnic groups, such as black, indigenous, and people of color, low-income, teen mothers, LGBTQ, and people of size. There are legitimate and substantial risks of falling prey to discrimination of all sorts, of being shoved out of the driver's seat, of receiving medical procedures and treatments you didn't want or consent to, and, ultimately, of feeling dehumanized and ending up with trauma and PTSD. There are many amazing blogs and books and support groups out there dealing with birth trauma.

Becoming thoroughly educated and informed throughout your pregnancy (even during the time you're planning a pregnancy), including the knowledge of your rights and how to defend them, will substantially shift the odds in favor of a safe and empowered birth experience.

My goal is to help you avoid birth trauma to begin with. Becoming thoroughly educated and informed throughout your pregnancy (even during the time you're planning a pregnancy), including the knowledge of your rights and how to defend them, will substantially shift the odds in favor of a safe and empowered birth experience.

A SAD, DISGRACEFUL STORY

Regarding the story I'm about to relay, I do so with permission from Kimberly Turbin, the courageous woman who took action for justice, and offered up incredible lessons in the process. Kimberly's story has been told many times in an effort to bring light to the rights of women during childbirth. My tender heart takes no comfort in the idea that it is often someone else's suffering that catalyzes our learning, but my pragmatic mind knows that we must indeed learn from both the experiences of others and our own histories. If we deny this, there is never a chance for growth. Let's learn from Kimberly's story.

The following is a transcript of dialogue and events taking place during an actual birth. In the room are Kimberly (the birthing woman), Kimberly's mother and sister (who is capturing the scene on video), Kimberly's friend, a labor and delivery nurse, and a doctor (obstetrician).

Definitions:
 ○ *Lithotomy position*: a supine position (flat on the back) of the body with the legs separated, flexed, and supported in raised stirrups, originally used for

---

lithotomy (removal of bladder or kidney stones) and later also for childbirth.

o *Perineum*: the space between the anus and the vaginal opening.

o *Episiotomy*: a surgical incision made at the opening of the vagina, through the perineum, involving skin and muscle.

Kimberly is lying in the lithotomy position on a hospital birthing bed. Only her lower body is visible. She is regionally anesthetized with an epidural. There is an internal bladder catheter emerging from her urethra, and a pulse oximeter attached to her toe. The nurse is on one side of Kimberly and her gaze is fixed on the monitor. Kimberly's friend is on the other side and is gently stroking Kimberly's arm with the back of her knuckles. The doctor is perched on a stool between Kimberly's legs and about three feet back, quietly waiting in a passive manner, as one would be if they were watching a performance or a TV show.

<u>Nurse:</u> Cinco de Mayo baby. It's going to come out with a sombrero. Just kidding. *(Laughs)*

It becomes apparent from the monitor that Kimberly is having a contraction.

<u>Nurse:</u> Ready? Take a nice deep breath.

Push him out. Go go go go. Push push push. Hard hard hard, just like that.
Go go go keep pushing, keep pushing. 6… 7… 8… 9… 10…

Good job. Again, come back up. Really hard. Push, push, push, push, go, go, go, go.
Just like that. Go! Go! Harder! Harder! Harder! Harder! Harder!
Go, go, go, go. And again, just like that. Push him out, come on.
Go, go, go. There he is. Go, go, go, keep pushing. Keep pushing. Keep pushing.
Hard, hard, hard, hard, hard. Go, go, go, go, go. Good job.
You have another one? Push, push, push, push, push, keep pushing.
Go, go, go, go, go, 7… 8… 9…and 10. Good job.

The doctor is now standing, unfolding a cloth while holding a pair of surgical scissors. The contraction ends and the doctor sits back down.

Kimberly's mother: Good job, babe.

Doctor: I'm going to do an episiotomy now.

Kimberly: What's up doctor?

Doctor *(pointing the scissors toward Kimberly)*: I said I'm going to do the episiotomy now.

Kimberly: What happened?

Nurse: So, he's saying he's going to have to do the episiotomy.

Kimberly: Why? We haven't even tried.

Doctor: *(pointing the scissors at her vagina as he speaks)* Kimberly, you are pushing, baby's head comes out and doesn't come out because there is no space here to come out. Ok? *(Forming circular shapes with his fingers...)* Baby's head about that big and your vagina is only that much. Ok?

Kimberly: *(talking as the doctor is demonstrating the size of the baby's head and her vagina)* So we're gonna try? We're gonna try?

Kimberly's mother: *(in Spanish)* He can't keep playing around! The baby has to come out.

Kimberly: Why can't we just try?

Doctor: Try? You're trying all the time and it doesn't come out. And if it comes out it's gonna rip the butt hole down clean. Ok?

Kimberly's mother: *(in Spanish)* Mm-hmm. Yes. It is true... that is what happened to Auntie R...

Kimberly's friend: You know sweetheart, you're not gonna feel it. Remember? And you have the epidural.

Nurse: Ok. Take a nice deep breath. And push, push, push. And push.

Kimberly's mother *(in Spanish)*: She says she wants for the baby to come out but the baby is not coming.

Nurse: 1...2...3...4...5...6...7...8...9... Keep going, keep going, Ok, good job. Nice deep breath. Push hard, hard, hard! Go, go, go, keep going. You're doing it.

Kimberly's friend and nurse are now verbally encouraging and cueing her together. There's a palpable crescendo in the room as the contractions come and it becomes apparent that something is about to occur.

Nurse and friend: Again, deep breath and again. Push hard, hard, hard. Push hard, hard, hard, keep going, keep going, keep going. Hard, hard, hard. Go, go, go, go, go.

The doctor comes closer, tosses the cloth on the lower portion of Kimberly's belly, just above the perineum with his left hand, as his right hand, holding the scissors, comes closer to Kimberly's genitals.

Kimberly: *(crying out)* No! Don't cut me!

Kimberly's mother: *(in Spanish)* Ok Kimberly! He has to do his job.

Doctor: *(turns slightly toward mother waving the scissors)* You tell 'em. I have to do it. Next time I'm gonna…

Kimberly's mother: Yes, I told her, I told her. I am her mother. I told her.

Kimberly: *(Crying with desperation)* Why? No!

Doctor: *(getting visibly frustrated and angry)* What do you mean "why"? That's *my* reason. I am the director here. Ok?

Kimberly: *(trying to be calm)* But why can't we try?

Doctor: *(mocking and gesticulating)* Why can't I do it? You can go home and do it. You go to Kentucky.

Kimberly: Can't we just…

<u>Kimberly's mother:</u> Nooo, Kimberly, you cannot fight with the doctor. Just do it doctor. Don't worry.

Kimberly and the nurse and friend are talking softly. It sounds like one of them is saying, "Sweetie, you're just really small." Kimberly is quietly pleading.

<u>Kimberly's mother:</u> Just do it doctor. Don't worry about it. She's…

Waiting for the next contraction, the doctor swabs the vaginal area and perineum with an anti-bacterial solution. The nurse is still softly trying to explain to Kimberly why this is necessary.

<u>Kimberly's mother:</u> *(in Spanish)* It is difficult for him, even if he tries, he doesn't have enough space and it is starting to "break".

The doctor is waiting for the next contraction with his left hand casually crossed over his right hand, holding the scissor.

<u>Nurse:</u> *(talking to Kimberly)* If you rip, you'll rip more than a cut and it's a lot more pain too.

<u>Kimberly's mother:</u> *(in Spanish)* It's nothing, "all that" will shrink back again.

<u>Nurse:</u> He said it's only an inch. An inch isn't that bad. Do you want to see an inch again?

The doctor turns around and grabs another cloth, unfolds it as the contraction starts.

<u>Kimberly:</u> I'm having a contraction.

<u>Nurse:</u> OK.

During the next few lines of dialogue from the nurse and Kimberly's mother, the doctor is methodically cutting Kimberly's perineum –
1 time
2 times
3 times
4 times
5 times
6 times
7 times
8 times
9 times
10 times
11 times
12 times.

<u>Nurse:</u> Push, push, push, push, push, push, push.

<u>Kimberly's mother:</u> It's fine – do it doctor.

<u>Nurse:</u> Keep pushing, keep pushing, keep pushing. Go, go, go, go.

Throughout, you hear the sound of the scissors cutting over and over and over again.

<u>Nurse:</u> Good job, good job, good job.

<u>Kimberly's mother:</u> *(in Spanish)* It's coming now!

Nurse: OK, and relax. And a nice deep breath.

Doctor is still cutting. Kimberly inhales and starts pushing again.

Nurse: Push and go, go, go, go, go, go, go.

The doctor is still cutting.

Kimberly's mother: *(in Spanish)* That's it. The baby is coming out already!

Nurse: Nice job. Keep going, keep going. More, more, more, more, more. Relax.

Kimberly's mother: *(in Spanish)* He wouldn't have come out if the doctor didn't do what he did.

The doctor is finally done cutting. He places one of the cloths over the baby's head as it emerges.

Nurse: Head's going to come out. He's coming. Hard, hard, hard. Go, go, go.
Keep pushing, keep pushing. Keep going. Push, push, push.

Kimberly's mother: *(in Spanish)* Here he is! Look at the baby! Look!

Nurse: We have a head. Really good sweetie, we have a head!

The doctor is now putting traction on the baby's head and neck to maneuver the shoulders.

Nurse: Push hard. Go, go, go. Hard, hard, hard, hard. There you go – he's almost out.

Kimberly's mother: Oh my god.

Nurse: Nice deep breath. Push really hard.

Kimberly's mother: (in Spanish) He's so beautiful!

Nurse: He's right there! Look! He's coming!

Kimberly's mother: (in Spanish) That's it. He's out! All white! Look! Oh, he is so cute. That is it daughter. He wouldn't have come out otherwise. He's very big.

The baby is finally given to Kimberly after 25 seconds of suctioning.

When Kimberly Turbin found out she was pregnant, she was excited. She was living in Chicago at the time and chose to move back to California to be closer to her family. She selected El Proyecto Del Barrio, a non-profit community health center, for her prenatal care, as this clinic's particular location was a convenient distance from her home. Kimberly's care was covered by Medi-Cal, California's state-run and funded Medicaid program. Although Kimberly was from the US, the majority of patients at El Proyecto Del Barrio were immigrants, and English was their second language.

She had an uneventful pregnancy, without even so much as nausea. No reason, at the time, to presume she would encounter any unusual circumstances during labor. Although she scanned YouTube videos and watched Ricki Lake's and Abby Epstein's documentary *The Business of Being Born*, which examines the ways that the American health care system approaches childbirth, she never felt compelled to further investigate her ability to advocate throughout the process, for her familial frame of reference posted no red flags. Kimberly explained, "Naturally, I didn't really ask anybody advice, or about what to do or not to do because there was nothing wrong with me and I never heard (about) my mom having any issue giving birth." As an eight-year-old she was present when her mom gave birth to her sister. "I just remember that the doctor was helping her. He actually worked with her while giving birth."

Her prenatal visits were routine, with 100% of her care being administered by various nurse practitioners. The doctors who would attend births would only interact with those women who had particular medical issues. For the most part, there was no relationship forged or opportunity to communicate directly with an obstetrician until the very end of pregnancy. Providers gleaned their information from the contents of the patients' charts.

The day before Kimberly reached 38 weeks, she met the doctor who would turn out to be the attending physician at her birth at Tarzana Providence Medical Center. According to Kimberly, he never looked her in the face during this visit. The very next day she went into labor.

During labor Kimberly made one thing clear. She told her caregivers, "I don't care what you do to me. I just need to know what you're doing before you do it." Of course, she did indeed care what was done to her, but her highest level of intention was to retain some semblance of control; to avoid, at all costs, any sort of perceived surprise attack, for she had endured her share of surprise attacks and significant, lingering trauma from past sexual assaults. The nurses were aware of her rape history, and yet there were no measures taken to mitigate a post-traumatic experience, aside from dispensing "a pill to calm her down" during labor. There was no prenatal counseling, no discussions providing informed consent, and no reassurance that measures would be taken to protect her sense of safety throughout the birth process, even though it is well established that past sexual abuse is often very triggering for victims during birth and commonly elicits deep feelings of fear. Kimberly didn't focus on this, for, again, she couldn't imagine anything going "wrong" when her pregnancy itself was unremarkable, and distress during birth was generally an unfamiliar concept to her. She bore no assumption that the devastation she experienced in her past would be cause for concern during labor and birth as long as she firmly communicated her simple two-line, non-negotiable requirement.

Sadly, Kimberly was mistaken in her expectations. Believing that control could be acquired and secured through simple, distinct communication, was naïve. Just as she had been ambushed before, another human's dangerous arrogance and deceit would strip her of control yet again. "I just remember thinking that I was being assaulted," she said. "I knew I was being assaulted because I could feel it… like I was being raped in front of everybody and nobody was noticing it… I was just scared of getting cut. I know I didn't need it. I know my body and I know I just didn't need it, so that's why I was saying 'no, don't cut me'. And I was scared to get an episiotomy because I'm scared of anyone going near my vagina, period… I'm terrified because of all the experiences that I've had. It's another guy forcing himself… to do something to my body that I just don't want done. It was just like getting raped."

How could that happen in a medical setting, where providers work from the foundation of "first do no harm" and the universal

145

assumption is that the hospital is a place filled with people who will take care of us, heal us and not hurt us, who want the best for those they serve? The reality is that as inconceivable as it might seem, it does happen, and it happened to Kimberly, who, unwittingly, became a victim of obstetric violence. With utter disregard for her rights as a birthing person, not to mention a human being, and despite her clear directive not to be cut, and her concise pleas to try to continue birthing her baby without an episiotomy, she was entirely ignored. Her demands were dismissed as irrelevant.

Learn from this. Being naïve and ignorant is not a crime, but it can harm you. The intention of relaying Kimberly's story is to motivate you to seek care that is evidence-based from a compassionate provider who respects diversity and individuality, and to encourage you to find the strength to walk away from any doctor-patient relationship that does not offer this, or just intuitively feels troublesome in any way. It is to persuade you to know your rights in general, and more specifically, to know your rights way before you have your first contraction.

WHAT NOW?

○ Learn about your rights.

○ Learn about the evidence-based benefits and risks of as many birth procedures as possible.

○ Ask for copies of hospital consent forms in advance of arriving at the hospital in labor. Take time to read them through thoroughly. Give yourself the opportunity to ask questions. Make notations and edits as you see fit, before signing.

○ It is difficult to watch, but if you feel it would be helpful to visualize Kimberly's experience, her YouTube video can be found here: youtube.com/watch?v=ICfXxtoAN-I

Thoughts and Actions

_____

_____

_____

_____

_____

_____

_____

_____

_____

_____

_____

Chapter 8

PAIN, MEET PURPOSE

"Birth isn't something we suffer, but something we actively do and exult in."

– SHEILA KITZINGER

What if, instead of going through labor, you went to sleep one night and woke up the following morning with a baby next to you? Before you scramble to figure out how to sign up for this theoretical fairytale, let's dissect what that would mean. Yes, it would mean no pain - and pain sucks. So, there's that. It would also cut down on anxiety since you wouldn't have to prepare or plan or think about pretty much anything at all. There would be no labor bag with snuggly socks and essential oils and massage tools; no need for deep connections with other moms and moms-to-be to exchange guidance and support; no late-night discussions with your partner, excitedly imagining how your story would unfold. No build-up, no process, nothing to recount other than, "I rolled over, and there he was!" No story to speak of.

Still want to pass on labor? Some of you may be saying, "No way", while others may be thinking, "Heck yeah, that all sounds good to me." I absolutely respect where you're coming from, no matter which team you're on. Regardless, I have lots more to share on this topic.

Your aversion to pain may not be the only reason why the little fable I offered up seems appealing to you, at least in part. There is no shortage of aversions to labor and the frightening assumptions one can invent in anticipation of giving birth. But let's just stay with pain, since it's a biggie.

PHYSICAL ASSOCIATION WITH PAIN

Pain serves a purpose. Physically, it relays signals that can shield us from instant harm, or further injury. The only reason you pull your hand back from a hot pan as quickly as you do is because of the immediate sensation of pain. Think about the end result if you didn't feel that pain and you allowed your hand to linger for a while. There's no denying that pain is unpleasant, but there are some very cool things that happen when you feel pain in labor. Your birthing body has a special wisdom.

Many of your hormones are part of an exquisite symphony during pregnancy, labor, birth, and postpartum, including the oxytocin that causes painful contractions and the endorphins that are released as nature's painkillers to help you manage the pain of those contractions. In order to assist your hormones in carrying out their duties, you might seek to master a cooperative control during labor, in which you observe and collaborate with the workings of your body, allowing the "musicians" to do their job. Interfering with the natural orchestration does not help, and can in fact be detrimental. Birth under medical management is like a group of spectators or concert organizers (care providers), who may have studied and practiced music for years, walking onto the stage, pushing aside the conductor (your hormones) and taking over the concerto. They wave their batons (medical interventions), attempting to bring together the flutes and the violins and dozens of other instruments to create the perfect melodies and harmonies (cervical dilation, baby's rotation and descent, etc.) but, with all their knowledge of music, they do not possess the skills of the conductor. They do not fully understand the nuances of this collaboration (the mysterious and unique qualities of each birth). At best, they can use their ability to keep the melodies going (labor progressing), coaxing out pieces of the composition, sometimes being lucky enough to make it to the final notes (birth) without being out of tune (some level of distress). In spite of the finish however, the musicians and instruments will never be in flow (labor will be forced). There will be no feel to the music, and it is highly probable that the arrangement will fall apart.

Of course, if an instrument needs tuning, and possibly in other uncommon circumstances, it would be justified to have collaborators on the stage, but only for isolated duties, and not as the norm. It would be like saying that, as a rule, the conductor is far less qualified and competent than the technicians and spectators. When you mess with your hormones, either by imposing superfluous medical interventions, or by fighting against the natural process of power and pain, you run the very high risk

THE ULTIMATE BIRTH EXPERIENCE

of ending up in a place you don't want to be. I suggest you hang a "Do Not Disturb" sign, both literally on the door of your labor room, and figuratively on the "doors" of your body and mind. Assuming there are no complications requiring necessary medical intervention, and you are working with your body to facilitate the progress of labor, your hormones can be trusted and should be greatly appreciated for the work they are doing on your behalf, and for your baby, even when that includes pain.

Pain triggers intuitive actions for comfort that are the same actions influencing the mechanics and progress of birth. Although you can learn about and reference different positions during labor, and those supporting you can make suggestions on which positions to take, it is fundamentally more effective to listen to your intuition. I speak from my own birthing experiences and those I've been lucky enough to be a part of, when I tell you that I've never known it to be easy and comfortable to manage the pain of contractions by lying in bed. In reality, the pain is much greater in a prone position than in an upright position. Movement also feels comforting, and most women, if not tethered to a bed, will naturally pace, sway, and rock during labor. It follows that employing gravity by choosing upright positions, and shifting your pelvis through movement, all for the intuitive purpose of pain relief, will encourage your cervix to open and your baby to wiggle their way through the pelvis.

Let's look at two ways in which labor pain can be managed with both the natural measures of positions and movement plus an epidural, and how one is more favorable than the other.

Mary goes into labor and mostly stays in bed or sits on the couch. After a couple of hours, she leaves for the hospital. Once she is admitted, she gets right into the hospital bed and

152

asks for an epidural. Her contractions have worked on their own to open her cervix to about 3 centimeters at this point. Once the epidural takes effect, Mary continues to lie, either on her left or right side, with no movement. Hours pass and there is no change to her cervix. She is relaxed and her uterus is relaxed. Her hormones, which might have kept working with her support, are no match for the anesthesia. Pitocin is started in an effort to augment her ineffective natural hormones. Her amniotic sac is also artificially broken. Her cervix dilates another 2 centimeters but her baby has not moved down. After several hours with no change, a C-section is performed.

Jane goes into labor and mixes up periods of rest and periods of gentle movement. She stays at home for several hours as her contractions continue to get longer, stronger, and closer together. She walks slowly in between contractions and then either gets into a "slow dance" position with her partner, swaying back and forth, or lays her upper body over a "birth ball" while on her knees, rocking her hips from side to side. Once she arrives at the hospital, she continues laboring out of bed, as she did at home, also standing in the shower and pacing around the room. Her cervix gradually dilates to 6 centimeters and her baby continues to descend further down into her pelvis, but after 3 hours with no change, hardly any sleep for 2 days prior, due to consistent practice contractions, and a total of 16 hours in labor, she is feeling exhausted and unable to manage the pain, even with all the tools in the Natural Bag. She chooses to get an epidural. She rests. Her body rests. Her contractions become more effective now that she is not stressed and subconsciously fighting the pain. When she has regrouped and gained some energy, she gets on her knees in bed, with the help of her nurse, and she leans over the birth ball, rocking her hips, which encourages the baby to keep moving down. Little by little the epidural medication is reduced, she begins to feel the urge to push, and within an hour, she gives birth, vaginally.

Mary did not see pain as purposeful. She didn't respond to her pain with positions and movements that would have offered some relief while, simultaneously, advancing her labor. Instead of listening to and working with her body, she walked into her labor pulling things out of the Medical Bag while neglecting her Natural Bag. Pain was not a prompt for her. It was something to be eradicated as quickly as possible. She denied her hormones the support they needed, and quickly subdued them.

Getting an epidural because you've been in labor for days, with no sleep, focusing every bit of your energy on dealing with the pain, after availing yourself of multiple tools from the no-risk Natural Bag, is not the same as viewing an epidural as your birthright, believing that you must get it at the earliest possible time in your labor, without assessing your ability to manage pain using those tools, or even knowing they exist.

Jane reacted to her pain with comfort measures that reinforced the work of her hormones. In response, her oxytocin initiated and enhanced her contractions. Gravity helped as well. Her contractions effectively opened her cervix and accelerated the passage of her baby through her pelvis. Because of her individual circumstances, she wisely assessed that she needed the epidural to rally, rest, and restore her strength and stamina. She listened to her body and her body rewarded her.

Yes, pain is purposeful, but it's also another "P" word: it's personal, like every other part of your birth. Getting an epidural because you've been in labor for days, with no sleep, focusing every bit of your energy on dealing with the pain, after availing yourself of multiple tools from the no-risk Natural Bag, is not the same as viewing an epidural as your birthright, believing that you must get it at the earliest possible time in your labor, without assessing your ability to manage pain using those tools, or even knowing they exist. At the end of the day, your decision to choose an epidural or not should 100% be acknowledged, respected, and supported. I simply offer an alternative viewpoint around labor pain, so that you appreciate its function and all of the benefits of the hormones at its core, and you recognize the many effective options for managing it. Passively and mechanically suppressing labor pain and disturbing the mission of your hormones can lead to greater challenges, and unexpected, unwanted consequences.

MENTAL ASSOCIATION WITH PAIN

The physical connection to pain's purpose is impressive. The mental relationship is equally as compelling.

Pain is part of the difficult, challenging, meaningful work that is birth. It is a piece of the tremendously complex, intense process of bringing forth life, packed with the extreme energy that precedes euphoria. Your confidence in either managing pain naturally or weighing the benefits and risks of pain medication to arrive at a well-thought-out choice, greatly increases the chance of an uncomplicated, safe birth.

THE ULTIMATE BIRTH EXPERIENCE

One of the core components of achieving your ultimate birth experience, and a theme we've been discussing throughout, is control. There is a common judgment that to be anything but a perfectly quiet, subdued bystander of your own labor, is unrefined. There is an underlying perception of dignity if you are sitting or lying in bed, attentively following protocols, and continuously able to interact. Getting on all fours, or squatting while naked, moaning and crying, is best left for the more primitive, "crunchy" crowd. Sadly, the ubiquitous view of being in control is actually the opposite of being in control. Don't misunderstand. You don't *have* to strip down and howl like a wolf, but, for sure, a woman who is so tuned into her needs and fully working with her labor is the one who defines dignity and control.

We may stand upright, have more well-developed brains, and use complex language, but humans are animals all the same, and although our higher intellect enables us to be the dominant species on Earth, denying our basic instincts can fail us. There are times, during labor and birth in particular, when allowing our natural mental and physical drives to take the lead is favorable. Control cannot be part of your experience if you don't surrender to your physiological responses, if you have no idea how to manage the pain of labor, if you need to, from the start, defer to someone else's idea of what you should be doing and how you should be behaving, and if you rely on them to handle your pain and expedite your labor.

It's also easy to associate pain with illness. Most of the time when we feel pain, something is wrong (even though it can still be the perfect indicator and motivator to do something that will cause healing and recovery.) Labor pain is not associated with illness though. The pain you will experience in childbirth comes directly from the muscular contracting (squeezing and tightening) of the uterus, the opening or dilating of the cervix (the neck of the uterus) and the stretching of the tissues in the vagina. This all must happen as part of the process of giving birth. One of the most meaningful provisions you should expect during your labor is that of reassurance. To be reminded throughout your labor that all is as it should be, that your pain is intentional, functional, and *good*, can instill feelings of comfort and a strong sense of will. You may think this won't be all that effective – but I assure you, it can make the difference between being overtaken by the storm or steering through it. With the help of your team, tap into your mind. Right now, in preparation for the day you go into labor, modify your thoughts and beliefs about pain, and then carry those new, healthy insights with you throughout your labor. Your mental state is, undeniably, as powerful as your physical condition.

Unless pain as part of the birthing process is perceived as necessary and significant, you will view yourself and be treated by others as a victim in need of rescuing, as opposed to a warrior in need of support.

Ina May Gaskin, an American midwife who has been described as "the mother of authentic midwifery" wrote in *Birth Matters:*

"One of the downfalls of our excessively comfortable society is the idea that pain is a bad thing to be avoided at all costs. We have built great pharmaceutical empires bent on masking, subduing and eradicating pain, even emotional pain, from our lives. We are taught to view pain as an enemy, not a teacher. But pain is the right hand of growth and transformation."

Unless pain as part of the birthing process is perceived as necessary and significant, you will view yourself and be treated by others as a victim in need of rescuing, as opposed to a warrior in need of support.

YOUR PERSONAL RELATIONSHIP WITH PAIN

Your understanding of the purpose behind labor pain will be helpful as you prepare for birth, and I hope you are beginning to accept and embrace the value, if not exactly getting excited over the prospect!

When I was pregnant with my first child, I couldn't understand why anyone would feel it was worthwhile to tolerate labor pain if, thanks to modern medicine, you could flip a switch and turn that pain off. Unlike many who shared, and still share that view, I didn't resist the idea of birth. I wasn't fearful or anxious about the birth process. On the contrary, I was that annoying woman who had easy pregnancies and marveled at just how big my belly could get! I longed for the day I'd go into labor, envisioning all of the tiny and grand moments from start to finish. Pain seemed like an interference, an irritating pest that would get in the way of my experience. I didn't know enough about birth and never considered how working through the pain, with the love and support of my husband, could add another dimension to my experience, and offer a chance for substantial personal growth.

In no way does my own epiphany translate into some revelation I think you should have. I am me and you are you. My only objective is to impart a balanced perspective by way of information you may never have known. I want you to understand the way your body works during labor and birth. I want you to see yourself as a capable person whose anatomy is designed for the purpose of giving birth. It is not a temperamental, unpredictable structure of arbitrary mechanisms. Not everything works perfectly every time, including birth, but there is an ancient reproductive system that lives inside of you. Pain is part of that system. To see it merely as an inconvenience you have no interest in experiencing, is to marginalize your remarkable body. It is to reduce it to that of a robot, a childbearing machine. Even if you believe that women feel pain in childbirth as some hand-me-down punishment, I still defend the physical and mental purpose in that pain.

Reverse engineer the process. Work backwards in your imagination from the point at which you have given birth and can reflect on your story. Did you put into practice your knowledge around dealing with labor pain? Did you show everyone around you what was helpful, merely by your actions, and did you tell them how to support you? If you chose to reach into the Medical Bag, were you able to make decisions about medication to help manage your pain because you understood the benefits for you in that unique moment in time? Empowerment comes from all of this. Respect your body. Respect your ability.

Similar to the implausible idea of waking up to find your baby lying next to you, having had no labor or memory of giving birth, is the absurd concept of a marathon runner or triathlete who receives their medal in the mail without ever going through the race and crossing the finish line. But if we linger in the make-believe for a moment, we can immediately recognize the tragic absence of so many transformational opportunities. I've asked athletes what mental changes and what lasting, life-enhancing benefits they felt they achieved along their travels to the finish line. Simply enduring the journey to, and on, "race day", with all of its challenges, was one discovery. There was the capacity to overcome fear, obstacles, and disappointments, and to remain committed to achieving something that was extremely difficult. They came away feeling that they had found things out about themselves they never knew existed, like the strength of their passion and resolution. They experienced enormous physical pain and found a way to fight past it by mastering their minds and harnessing their deepest motives. Never quitting. Never having regrets.

Labor will be your race day. Find the purpose in your pain.

WHAT NOW?

○ Break ties with anyone who is scaring you about birth. Surround yourself with people who will be honest, realistic, and encouraging. Be with those who believe in you and value the birth process.

○ Go as deeply as possible into learning about both natural comfort measures and medical options for managing labor pain.

○ Communicate with your birth team. Let each person know how you want to be supported, specifically when it comes to pain management.

Thoughts and Actions

Chapter 9

THE VBAC VORTEX

"Sometimes you make the right decision, sometimes you make the decision right."

— PHIL MCGRAW

Your ultimate birth experience is not necessarily synonymous with a natural, vaginal birth. It certainly doesn't equate with an intervention-free birth at all costs. There are very appropriate and beneficial reasons to embrace medical procedures. Giving birth via C-section, even if you are fiercely opposed to this option and you're doing all you can to avoid it, can sometimes end up being favorable from a medical standpoint and when accounting for personal considerations. Be that as it may, when the dream is not realized, it is common to feel defeated. Many women who have gone through this will believe that their bodies have failed them.

If this was your experience, it is possible that you were left with a sense of anguish over an unintended C-section. Whether Mother Nature pulled the rug out from under you or you were mistreated in some way, the physical and psychological impact can cause you to feel broken. You have opportunities to heal. One remedy could be the realized goal of having a vaginal birth after Cesarean (VBAC) if you choose to have another baby. If this scenario speaks to you and you would like to consider a VBAC but feel overwhelmed by conflicting messages and you don't know where to start, then this chapter is for you.

As with all of the very personal decisions you will make, you should never be pressured in any direction. You may be blasted with opinions and advice. There will be those who will endorse VBAC with compelling enthusiasm, and those who will affirm the virtues of a repeat Cesarean with the same zeal. Seeking guidance from those you trust may be helpful. In the end, you are entitled to figure out what is best for you.

The fact remains that high rates of surgical births have, on one hand, normalized C-sections, and on the other, created a tribe of mothers who long for a different birth experience. Sadly, many who hope for a VBAC have been told it is selfish and unrealistic to even consider an alternative birth method to a repeat Cesarean. My goal is to empower and inform you to make a decision that is best for *you* and to have the courage, through knowledge, to vocalize your decision and surround yourself with the people and places that will support that decision.

SORTING THROUGH FACTS AND MYTHS

As with many beliefs surrounding birth, VBAC is a topic with an underpinning of judgments and theories. If you so much as broach the subject with those operating from a place of fear, it is likely you'll be faced with a reaction suggesting you just proclaimed your desire to sail into the Bermuda Triangle during a hurricane. This fear is culturally pervasive and can lead to sweeping generalizations in which all people and all situations need to fit neatly into a prescribed, secure box. We see this in the way birth is perceived by many practitioners, institutions and much of the birthing population. Should you be considering a VBAC, it is not okay to be treated as if you are out of line or out of your mind. You deserve to have a thoughtful, personalized conversation with your care provider.

VBAC, or more specifically TOLAC (Trial of Labor After Cesarean) is not without risks, just as ERCS (Elective Repeat Cesarean Section) is not without risks. For some, the actual and perceived risks of VBAC will be the greater influence during the decision-making process, while for others, the benefits will have more of an impact. To vehemently reject the option with absolute assertion that this is entirely dangerous and irrational is misleading and false. It shows a lack of awareness in general, and if it is a medical provider enforcing the veto, it also constitutes an omission of informed consent.

When choosing whether to plan for a VBAC or an ERCS, it can be helpful to look at what the research reveals. The gold standard to date for a comprehensive report, incorporating mountains of data, comes from the National Institute of Health Consensus Statement. (7) The NIH Consensus and State-of-the-Science Statement was created from the insights of a 15-member panel of healthcare professionals including representatives from the fields of obstetrics and gynecology, midwifery, maternal and fetal medicine, and more, plus the data from 20 other experts in pertinent fields.

Contained in the conclusions is the following:

Given the available evidence, trial of labor is a reasonable option for many pregnant women with one prior low transverse uterine incision.

When trial of labor and elective repeat Cesarean delivery are medically equivalent options, a shared decision-making process should be adopted and, whenever possible, the woman's preference should be honored.

Success of trial of labor is consistently high, ranging from 60 to 80 percent, whereas the risk of uterine rupture is low, at less than 1 percent.

It is wise to discuss the risks and benefits of trial of labor, vaginal birth, and repeat Cesarean with a trusted care provider who relies on the information included in this report and values the shared decision-making process. It is important to know the evidence, and it is equally important to understand the limitations of this evidence.

Even if you are someone who does not feel a strong personal commitment to a VBAC, your care provider may still recommend a trial of labor if you're intending to have more than one child after your previous C-section. Multiple C-sections increase the risk of placenta previa (when the placenta partially or completely covers the cervix) and placenta accreta (when the placenta attaches too deeply into the uterine wall), in addition to other risks including long-term health implications. Of course, you still have the final say and your doctor or midwife should always be sensitive to that end, but within that framework of respect, recommending a VBAC if your plan is for future pregnancies, would be appropriate.

Ultimately, I would urge you to keep in mind that there are no guarantees – that this is not open and shut, just as any birth, under any circumstances, including a first birth with no complications, does not embody 100% assurance of absolute safety and a specific result. Although there are screening tools that attempt to forecast risk and can be used with the aim to predict an outcome, it remains difficult to know who will have a successful VBAC and who will experience rare adverse outcomes from either VBAC *or* ERCS.

AGE AND VBAC

Oftentimes women are denied the option of a trial of labor for a VBAC based on age. Many care providers will cite the evidence pertaining to a lower VBAC success rate and higher incidence of uterine rupture for women 35 and older. Please take note of what the evidence actually shows: The likelihood of vaginal birth is "slightly lower" and the evidence for risk of uterine rupture is "conflicting – *may be* slightly higher".(8) This hardly substantiates the degree of danger that would influence a practitioner's advice against a trial of labor.

Moreover, in line with the entire theme of *The Ultimate Birth Experience*, every birth, every birthing person, and every aspect of every situation is unique. As pointed out earlier, no matter

A woman over 35 who smokes, ignores her health, and leads a stressful life is not equivalent to a woman over 35 who does not smoke, focuses on her health, and manages her stress.

what the circumstances are, it is not possible to know, for sure, that a particular decision is going to lead to a particular outcome. Add to that the singular characteristics of the individual, and the difficulty in making predictions is reinforced. A woman over 35 who smokes, ignores her health, and leads a stressful life is not equivalent to a woman over 35 who does not smoke, focuses on her health, and manages her stress.

For certain, your age alone should not be the reason you decide to surrender your wishes for a VBAC.

THE VBAC CALCULATOR

There are resources that have been created called VBAC calculators that estimate the odds of having a successful VBAC. Certain values such as age, height, weight, body mass index, previous vaginal delivery, race and ethnicity are included.(9) Where some care providers will unconditionally rely on this calculator to support or oppose a VBAC, others will see it as a tool that has its place within a broader view. Instead of shutting down options and inciting self-doubt, they will include these calculations in the discussions they have with their patients, along with a holistic approach that allows for thoughtful consideration in the personal decision-making process.

Be wary of accepting advice based on statistics without the benefit of exploring all of the factors and possibilities. It can feel so scientific, so real and tangible, to be presented with a score, but it leaves out many essential components of an event that has both physiological and psychological influences and isn't as predictable as one might think.

If you are working with those who strongly believe in the worth and virtues of the VBAC calculator, the treatment you receive will be based, in part, on those beliefs, whether the results are encouraging or discouraging. This alone can change the course of what will eventually happen.

It just makes sense to partner with a birth team that values a more individualized approach, one in which you are counseled on the best evidence and general recommendations through informed choice discussions. There are providers who understand the limitations of VBAC calculators. They appreciate the unique characteristics of each woman, each pregnancy, and each birth. My commitment is to remind you of your control in finding such a provider.

PAST BIRTH EXPERIENCES

Another factor that is considered when determining the odds of a successful trial of labor leading to VBAC is the reason a woman had a C-section in her previous birth to begin with. If the C-section was done because the baby was in a breech position, the probability of achieving a VBAC is higher than if the C-section was the result of arrested dilation and descent, known as "failure to progress". As with relying on age, race and ethnicity in determining odds, there are gaps. If you have been led to believe that your odds of a VBAC are lower because you didn't dilate in your first birth (or any previous birth that led to a Cesarean), or because your baby never descended far enough, whether before or during pushing, it's important to assess the details of that past birth.

There are clear recommendations by ACOG (American College of Obstetricians and Gynecologists) for the Safe Prevention of the Primary Cesarean Delivery. (10)

Here is a paraphrased summary of some of these recommendations as they pertain to circumstances that could contribute to a failure to progress conclusion:

- The length of time in active labor should not be an indication for Cesarean delivery.
- Slow, but progressive labor should not be an indication for Cesarean delivery.
- One should not be considered to be in active labor until they are 6 centimeters dilated, and at that point Cesarean delivery for failure to progress should not be an indication unless their water has broken and they've been having adequate contractions for 4 hours, or they've had pitocin for 6 hours without dilating any further.
- Although 2-3 hours of pushing (depending on whether you've given birth before, or this is your first birth) is typically the maximum length of time designated before recommending a Cesarean delivery, longer durations may be appropriate on an individualized basis.

Certainly, from a medical standpoint, it seems wise to combine these recommendations with the comprehensive assessments of a skilled doctor or midwife. It is when these recommendations are disregarded that the question of an accurate diagnosis leading to a Cesarean delivery would be justifiable.

Similarly, it would be relevant to take a look back and evaluate the choices you personally made or didn't make that might have influenced the outcome of that birth. It's possible that you didn't have the necessary knowledge, and/or you were not being appropriately guided and supported, both of which could easily be amended this time around. As a simple reflective exercise, ask yourself:

- o   Did I consistently use gravity and move during labor?
- o   Did I use natural methods to expedite the progress of dilation before receiving medical interventions such as artificial rupture of membranes and pitocin, or did I experience those interventions as part of a routine protocol?
- o   Was I encouraged to get out of bed, use the shower, sit on or lean over a birth ball, change positions and use visualization?
- o   Was my birth team made up of people who believed in my ability to birth my baby vaginally and who supported me in every way possible to achieve that result?
- o   Did I get an epidural because I didn't know I had other options, or as an in-the-moment calculated strategy toward a vaginal birth?
- o   If the determination of failure to progress was made during the time I was pushing, had I tried several positions? Was I encouraged to use a squatting bar to push in a full squatting position?

If ACOG recommendations in your previous birth were not followed, and/or you answered "no" to many of those questions, then relying on the argument against VBAC now, due to a history of arrested dilation and descent, is not as straightforward as it appears to be. There's the possibility that the arrest might have been avoided or reversed, which validates your attempt for a VBAC. Bringing this to light may stir up some disappointment and regret, but I encourage you to focus on the positive, and on the present. This is an opportunity to use what you know to advocate for a safe trial of labor and an eventual VBAC, if that is what you want.

HOW COMMITTED ARE YOU?

Your mindset may just be the most influential determinant of your odds of having a successful VBAC. If you are frightened, not completely committed to the idea of a VBAC, not fully supported by your partner, other family members and care providers, and pressured into submitting to the standard list of routine interventions, you'll be up against many strikes from the start. On the other hand, a successful trial of labor leading to a VBAC is much more likely to be realized when you believe it's the right thing to do and when there is full and genuine support by the entire birth team. Are you going to walk into this with fear? Because fear on your part or your practitioner's part is going to change everything. You have to trust the birth process, and have faith that your body can do

> *Are you going to walk into this with fear? Because fear on your part or your practitioner's part is going to change everything. You have to trust the birth process, and have faith that your body can do this.*

this. You must tolerate being pregnant until your body and your baby indicate that it's time for labor, as opposed to begging for an induction because you're sick of being pregnant. Going into spontaneous labor, whenever possible, increases the odds of a successful VBAC.

Hoping and praying will not be enough to lead you to your goal – your VBAC goal, other birth-related goals, or any goal for that matter. There is work involved. The foundation of that work begins with your thoughts, your beliefs, and your will.

FINAL TAKEAWAY

You can get lost in the weeds and tumble down into rabbit holes. You can live in fear and be consumed by worry. But if VBAC is an option you want to pursue, then you should pursue it. It's likely that you'll be somewhere on the spectrum of having a pretty good shot to being a fabulous candidate. Your measurable circumstances have so many variables, and that's not even taking into account things like your attitude and dedication to the process that are not measurable. Even when relying on calculators, (which we know are imperfect tools), predicting only a moderate success rate doesn't mean you're not going to succeed. As one midwife put it, "It's a freakin' number." You have every right to *try*. Being labeled with a high or low probability of VBAC can be a self-fulfilling prophecy if it leads to doubt on your part or changes how you are cared for during labor, so work with those who will not project those labels.

No different than in any other pregnancy, the ingredients that go into the journey along the way toward planning a VBAC will be powerful sources of your ultimate birth experience. Having a vaginal birth after a Cesarean, especially a Cesarean that was the culmination of a traumatic birth, will be healing and victorious. But with the most committed mindset, thorough action steps toward the goal, and genuine, exhaustive support, your initial devastation, should a VBAC not be realized, will give way to acceptance and gratitude for all you've taken control of, and for the kind, faithful treatment you sought out and secured.

WHAT NOW?

○ Decide if a VBAC is important to you. Exploring the option may confirm what you've felt all along or it may change your initial feelings. Resist the urge to cave under the pressure of judgment. Be clear about your desires and dedication as you create and work toward your goals. It's the only way you'll reach them.

○ Choose a care provider who is aware of and advocates for the most current research supporting VBAC as a safe option for women who have had a previous C-section with an incision in the lower segment of the uterus. This should also be someone who trusts your ability to make informed decisions about your own care, who is not making recommendations based on concerns over liability and perceived risk, but rather, on evidence and the thoughtful, sensible interpretation of the data.

○ Seek out the hospitals that support VBAC. There are barriers that women face in gaining access to clinicians and facilities that are able and willing to offer TOLAC, so be certain that you are in a VBAC-friendly environment.

○ Spend time preparing. Read, take classes, and make sure your partner and other family members are educating themselves right alongside you so that they are as comfortable and committed as you are.

○ Join VBAC support groups. Connect with those on the same path as you, as well as those who have come before you and have navigated the choppy waters. This will offer the support and encouragement you need. Simply speaking with people in your inner circle, especially if they are repeating what they've heard or have been told, without evidence-based information provided by an open-minded resource, may confuse you even more.

Thoughts and Actions

Chapter 10

THE FOREVER MAGIC OF BIRTH

"Childbirth is an experience in a woman's life that holds the power to transform her forever."
— SUZANNE ARMS

There are limited opportunities with the power to peel away your layers to the very core of your soul, and reveal an exclusive, one-of-a-kind treasure map that can guide you through your life. Giving birth is one of those opportunities.

I imagine, being someone who is intrigued by designing your ultimate birth experience, you thoroughly and organically understand this. The idea of birth being mystical and sacred feels on point. Whether you've already given birth or not, you just know that there is magic at its center. You appreciate, so perfectly, how this will change you forever.

You also understand that you can't separate a cherished experience from the best experience. The required heart and soul you must put into the steps toward your dreams is, by definition, what makes it the best. Your thoughts, your beliefs, and your actions are what provide the power to determine your perception of the result – not the circumstances you can't govern.

How tragic that women are judged to be prioritizing the experience of giving birth over the outcome of a healthy baby, as if the experience is meaningless, and the two are disconnected; mutually exclusive. That is actually the theory: that endeavoring to honor birth as the greatest, most significant multi-faceted transformation in a person's life, somehow minimizes and devalues having a safe birth and a healthy baby. You can't separate the experience from the outcome. They are completely interrelated, both medically and emotionally. You happen to birth even more than birth happens to you. Or you can – and I hope you will.

An empowered birth holds the potential to restore the spirit of someone who has previously experienced heartbreak and grief during a past birth and otherwise. It can repair what is broken and nourish what is lacking. It can top off and add abundance to an already full and satisfied life.

Early on in my relationship with my husband, we talked about having a bunch of kids. At one point, he mentioned wanting to have five children, but that was before we had two, who were less than two years apart in age. And let's not forget about the mortgage and car payments. The realities of life pulled us both down to earth. I knew we'd probably decide to adjust our original plan. What I didn't know at the time was that my husband's thoughts around modifying our initial intentions were not in line with mine, but I would soon find out. I started to see how five children might not be in our future. I was content with the idea of three, and just assumed that's where we were heading – until one day, when it came up in conversation and I mentioned something about "when I would be pregnant again...", and he casually slipped in that he was fine with just having two. My heart sunk. I was honestly shocked. I absolutely assumed we'd have another baby. Although these were big decisions in their own right, we weren't talking about a vacation or a car. This was my life. That's how I saw it. I had so many deep feelings about having a third child but, in that moment, I couldn't articulate any of them. I just felt crushed. I didn't want to convince him. I didn't want to add to our family unless he was completely on board, and even that wouldn't have been enough. I wanted him to be as excited over the prospect and as committed to the significance as I was. I sat with the heaviness for a few days, secretly mourning the loss of my dream, trying to make sense of why this was such a blow. After all, we had two healthy children. It would not be the end of the world if I never got pregnant again and we remained a family of four. What I realized was that my anguish didn't come from a place of disappointment. I wasn't simply sad because I had expected we'd have another baby and now it looked like that wasn't going to happen. This was so much deeper. It was connected to what defined my values and how I determined what was worthwhile in life. Once I realized this, I wrote a letter – something I did, and still do often, when it feels too difficult to clearly communicate through overwhelming emotions.

At the root of my explanation as to why another pregnancy felt vital to me, why adding to our family was so fiercely important, was purely the fact that we *could*. My whole life I had longed for a sibling without disabilities. I ached for my brother to be normal, to lead a normal life, for us to have a normal relationship. I cried many tears over the suffering my parents endured. There was nothing I could do to change the circumstances.

Five months before my father would walk me down the aisle, I watched him die suddenly right in front of me. Once again, and at other less profound moments along my life's timeline, there was nothing I could do to control what was happening. But, to have another baby, to have a "big" family, to have more fulfillment, more joy, more goodness in my future – I *did*… we *did* have control over that. We *could* change the circumstances. Although the reasons not to have a third child were clamoring for our attention, not one could raise its voice above the crescendo in my heart that was screaming, "This is right. This is your life. This is the authority you have over your happiness. Go for it."

The next day I found a letter in reply, sitting on my pillow. I was heard. I was validated. I was understood. The depths of my desire to seize whatever control I had in this one go-around on the planet was appreciated, and eventually shared.

And so, with the drive to steer my own ship, mixed with the knowledge I had gained after the birth of my first two children, I created the most empowering birth experience possible. The end goal had been to expand our family, but it was the planning of this birth, and then every detail of how it would eventually develop (including having my children in the room as their baby sister was born) that generated the ultimate, lifelong dividends achieved by doing what it takes to manifest our destinies.

WHAT BIRTH TEACHES YOU

Resilience, bravery, and courage are not always the strengths you embody before giving birth, but they are the ones that are often forged and shaped through the process. Giving birth teaches perspective, balance and presence. What frightens many people also has the potential to build their confidence. As with other experiences that require great mental and physical effort, and come with challenges you must face, your birth experience will be an event you can draw upon to find the stamina, the fortitude, and the ability to adapt to stress and adversity when facing future challenges.

As with other experiences that require great mental and physical effort, and come with challenges you must face, your birth experience will be an event you can draw upon to find the stamina, the fortitude, and the ability to adapt to stress and adversity when facing future challenges.

You will be offered the chance to learn about, and to use the skills responsible for making high-stakes decisions, to have agency over your own choices, and to discover how to change course with relative ease when things don't go as expected.

Birth will lay the groundwork for living a life of autonomy and the belief in your competence. As one mom expressed, "I felt like if I could do that, then I could pretty much do anything. I felt so strong and capable and informed. I think a lot of those feelings stemmed from being able to make my own informed choices in pregnancy, labor and birth, and having those choices respected by my family and care providers. I made decisions and called the shots, and the midwives were there in case I needed emergency help. I was an active participant and authority in my babies' births. It was not something that just 'happened' to me."

If you've already given birth and your experience was not what you had hoped for, if you feel desensitized, cheated and angry, especially if you are filled with guilt and remorse, I say this to you as sincerely as possible: every life experience... *every single one*... is a gift. Some of these gifts are cleverly disguised as hardships, disappointments, and punishments. Your initial instinct will almost always be to fall victim, to be beaten down, to give up. I understand. But stop and ask yourself, "What is my goal?" Do you want to, ultimately, be happy or sad? If you could, would you choose to rise above or stay in this distressed state? There is a way out, and for different people, it requires different strategies. But the common starting point is always made up of two steps. One is to be kind to yourself – as genuinely kind as you'd be to another person in your same, exact place. Two is to open the gift and see it for what it is – a chance to turn it over and around, to shake it, to look at it through a magnifying glass, to inspect every detail, and to *use* it forevermore. Conjure it up, just as you would if your birth experience had been empowering, but in its own, distinctive way. Pull it apart and apply its pieces to your life. That can include a future birth, various relationships, and your role as a mother. Feelings of intimidation and the experience of being bullied should not be forgotten. They should be implemented.

You will never gain strength and confidence by pushing the experience away, letting it overtake you, or by ignoring the crappy emotions that surface. Stay conscious. Be fiercely aware of your past behavior, circumstances, and actions or inactions. Remain determined to create boundaries around that which threatens to bring you down, but hold its hand and drag it around with you wherever you go, so that it teaches you how to handle situations the way you want to, with the thoughts and beliefs that benefit you. History is the most powerful teacher. Sometimes it even has to repeat itself to offer reminders and further teaching. Embrace all that happens to you, in birth and otherwise, and implement it to craft your future self and to inspire your children to do the same.

CARING "TOO MUCH"

You don't wake up in the morning and say, "I'm not going to put anything on my schedule because I'm sure something's going to come up." You plan and you pivot.

That's the profound feature of birth and how it can influence every part of the rest of your life. There's no shame in declaring your intention to have a natural, vaginal birth only to end up with a C-section. Ask yourself:

- "Did I know what was going on?"
- "Did I retain my voice?"
- "Did I have a partnership with my caregivers and the other people on the team?"
- "Was I able to ask questions and get answers that I understood?"
- "Did I feel in control?"

So, yes, of course, if you are the person who values planning and preparing, who will nobly create a goal and move forward with force and determination to reach it, that is virtuous and worthwhile. However, if there is no "losing", no "second best" for you, no acceptance of working with that which is not necessarily in your control, you will go from natural disappointment to disabling devastation. Depending on how much you may need to shift, how dramatically nature may mess with your plan, and how much of a perfectionist you were to begin with, you will be sad, and you will need to grieve for those lost goals. You will, possibly, feel shame and disgrace for falling short of arriving at a preconceived place you assumed you would be. It is now time to redefine success. Use this most miraculous moment of pregnancy – of literally creating life – to interpret success in a new, and much more meaningful way. Shine the spotlight on all you are doing leading up to your birth that is setting the stage for achievement, because even without the final, longed-for outcome, you have so many reasons to hold your head high. The luck that comes along for the ride is not the substance of distinction. It's not what raises the bar and fosters proficiency for the rest of your life. In retrospect, focus on every drop of physical and mental effort you expended during your labor and recognize its connection to all the good in the end. Take a moment to think about what might have materialized if you *didn't* learn and advocate and carefully choose your team, if you *didn't* work with your body, and ask questions. Hold onto how you harnessed the control. Arrive at the place where you feel proud and confident. Always look forward, carrying that pride and confidence with you into every facet of your future.

NOT CARING ENOUGH

There will be women who have given birth who will say that this sounds like unicorns and rainbows; that birth is just an excruciating, gut-wrenching physical process you must go through to get your baby out; that the only transformation taking place is to your "scarred" body. Someone who was never surrounded by joyful birth stories, or never explored any of their deeper feelings about birth before and throughout their pregnancy, or someone who perceived a managed and regulated birth as the model for the highest standards of safety, would not have a reason to believe otherwise. They wouldn't think to draw upon their birth

Birth, represented by the stories we're told that shape our paradigms, and colored by our personal experiences, can have a tremendous influence on how we show up in the world. And for those who birth "on purpose", it almost always does.

experience when dealing with the challenges of being a new mom and other trials of life. Because they would have come from a place of indifference and then remained passive in their own experience, they might perceive you as being foolish for believing birth could be more than a flawed bodily function; a random, imperfect occurrence.

For anyone who regards every major life experience as simply a means to an end, I say, respectfully, that you are not living life to the fullest. I certainly don't believe that the way we view birth and the way we give birth are the only driving forces determining our senses of self-efficacy and levels of confidence, and our only opportunities to build resilience and courage. Nor do I suppose that we can't find empowerment and happiness in our lives in countless other ways. But birth, represented by the stories we're told that shape our paradigms, and colored by our personal experiences, can have a tremendous influence on how we show up in the world. And for those who birth "on purpose", it almost always does.

There are also those who have given birth who will tell you that they had intentions, that they had this sense that working toward a goal was worthwhile, and they believed they had some control. They didn't buy into the idea that birth is a haphazard series of random events. They "educated" themselves by reading some blogs and signing up for the hospital childbirth class. There was even a conversation that occurred at one of their prenatal visits where they told their doctor what their preferences were. But nothing went as planned, and therefore, "All of the effort you're putting into this 'ultimate birth experience'", they'll admonish, "is a waste of time."

The mistake that led to their unintended outcomes and subsequent cynicism, was the inadequate effort in becoming truly educated, and their lack of sufficient advocacy. They had the expectation that their wishes would be granted by reading here and there, taking a class that only yielded information on protocols, and then letting their caregivers know that "this" is what they wanted. Even if they had done a more thorough job of becoming informed and communicating with more clarity and strength, they, apparently, neglected to gain an understanding of how the ultimate birth experience can be realized without the entire plan materializing.

It is not enough to *want* anything – a natural birth without medication, no routine interventions, a vaginal birth, support during labor, informed consent, evidence-based care. You can't expect to get close to your actual wishes, or to extract any of the indirect character-building advantages throughout your labor by scanning fragments of information that may or may not be accurate and scientifically backed. It is improbable that you will have anything other than the standard "leave-everything-to-us-experience" if you don't actively assert your rights, or if you are planning to give birth in a hospital that strictly follows the medical management of labor model and has a 40% C-section rate. Same thing if you're shot down or placated during discussions with your medical care provider, but you insist on sticking around because, "It's just too hard to switch providers, especially toward the end." Hoping for the best is not a strategy for success.

CREATING A FAMILY

It is heartbreaking, disturbing, and downright pathetic that we've relegated birth to a series of medical procedures, ostensibly, to guarantee a healthy outcome. We are humans acting like robots. This cultural concept dismisses the fact that birth is the continuum of our descendants and the progression of our futures. It abandons the strongest, most compelling dynamic of birth... that it is the creation of a family, and, if nurtured as such, can serve to change and enrich the entire life of parent and child.

This experience is not simply the birth of your baby. It is *your* birth into a brand new identity, one that if supported, revered and nurtured as it should be, has endless potential for you as an individual and for your family.

THE EFFECT OF YOUR BIRTH, POSTPARTUM

Paying attention to your wellness and wellbeing during your pregnancy – to your physical health, through exercise, nutrition and stress-management, to your relationships, especially with your partner, to your community, by engaging with other pregnant moms and moms who have gone through their own empowering experiences, will all set you up for the ultimate *postpartum* experience. We typically define "postpartum" as the time just after giving birth – maybe a few weeks to a few months. This is the acute time of transformation, and all of that attention you gave to your physical and mental health throughout pregnancy will carry over into this brief phase. But, really, "postpartum" is your whole life as a mother after you give birth, which makes the effects of your birth experience enduring.

Every "t" crossed and every "i" dotted along your pregnancy and birth journey, every ounce of effort you put into doing your best, into managing the circumstances that are in your control while building strength and resolve when faced with challenges, will be the gifts that keep on giving.

There will be another person who is equally as influenced by your empowering birth experience. All that you do will, indirectly, have an effect on the health and wellness of your baby - first, in a distinctly physical way, and then, as you enter into parenthood, in your parent-child relationship. Every step you take toward a conscious, gentle birth will bring your baby into this world in a conscious, gentle way.

You may not think that your newborn infant will be touched by your stress, self-doubt or lack of confidence, but we, as humans, absorb the energy that is around us, regardless of our age. Although a baby's brain may not be developed enough to understand the subtleties of language as we do, that brand new nervous system is equally as sensitive to the intangible energy he or she is exposed to. Touching and nurturing a baby can go a long way toward neutralizing the stress they may, on occasion, sense from unavoidable situations, but wouldn't it be amazing if the very first, most significant experience of being born could be filled with love and triumph? This can be the case whether you give birth naturally in a tub in your home, or in a hospital on an operating room table. Value your own growth and transformation toward this end, so that your birth is victorious, and your sweet baby takes that in from the very start of their life.

I LEAVE YOU WITH THIS

So much of your life will take place after you have given birth. Your birth experience or experiences will be collections of memories and stories you tell. The only time to shape those memories and stories is now. It is worth it. Whatever your heart and your intuition is telling you to do, it is worth it. It may be emotionally difficult. It may, at times, fill you with aching self-doubt. It may be so confusing and exhausting that you'll want to give up and fall into line with the masses just to take a break from the effort required to maintain your autonomy. Please don't. You deserve to live with sincerity, honoring your truth and all that is most important to you. You are so very entitled to a life without regret, but only you can make that happen by your actions in the here and now. You will reach a tipping point where your conviction outweighs your uncertainty. I promise.

Consistently surround yourself with those who honor and encourage your individuality. Distance yourself from those who evoke feelings of defensiveness. Do everything in your power not to wake up one day, whether just after you gave birth or many years later, wondering why you didn't seek to know, or take a different path once you did. Discover who you are, right now, and be brave in the pursuit of what you want.

Focusing on your birth experience will never be a waste of time. Focusing on your birth experience will open doors you didn't know existed. It will level the playing field and afford you the ability to be the master of your own life. It will, in the end, reduce anxiety and heighten your belief in yourself. Those you interact with and their attitudes about birth, the way you are treated by the most influential people in your life during your pregnancy, what you know and how you obtain that knowledge, can make the difference between a safe and a compromised pregnancy and birth, and between deep satisfaction with yourself and feelings of intense remorse.

Bronnie Ware, Australian author, songwriter and motivational speaker, is best known for her writings about the top deathbed regrets she heard during her time as a palliative care provider. She has listed and described these regrets in her book, *The Top Five Regrets of the Dying*. The number one regret disclosed was:

"I wish I'd had the courage to live a life true to myself, not the life others expected of me."

The magic is in having the courage, at a pivotal juncture in your life – a time of great hope and eager anticipation for what is to come – to find out who you are, and then never, under any circumstances, forsake your truth.

This is where I believe the magic lies, in birth as in life. Not in expecting absolute assurances, or in getting it "right". Not in remaining complacent and staying under the radar so as not to disturb the status quo. Not in ignoring the vibrant uniqueness that is you because of another's views or pressure or judgment. The magic is in having the courage, at a pivotal juncture in your life – a time of great hope and eager anticipation for what is to come – to find out who you are, and then never, under any circumstances, forsake your truth.

When you operate from your genuine core, refusing to be knocked off balance by the misleading idea that truth resides in numbers, you will always be rewarded at the highest level. Having your baby in the way others expect you to have your baby, just like living your entire life to the same end, will not shield you from the ridicule you are trying to avoid, and even if it did – at what cost?

Beautiful, empowered, birthing woman, listen to your innate wisdom. Make your own choices, design your own journey, and take control of your own fate. Set the stage for the rest of your life and set the examples you want your children to emulate and embody for the rest of theirs. Walk courageously into the experience of a lifetime - your ultimate birth experience.

APPRECIATION

When my friend Karen Alpert was pregnant for the first time, after I had already given birth twice, I could not understand why she was planning to attempt a birth without medication and other interventions. As enthralled as I was with having babies, my own birth experiences did not include the meaningful planning she was executing. She was much wiser and more informed than I was. I questioned why she would want to be a martyr (which she gracefully dismissed). And yet, I still had this burning desire to be part of birth. I had a certain vision of helping women through labor and would talk about this fantasy all the time. With a giant dose of poetic justice, it was Karen who came back from a childbirth class announcing that there was an actual profession that fit my description. "You want to be a 'birth doula'!" she exclaimed. I imagine I would have, eventually, found my way to where I am, but I'm in love with this story of how it all began. Tucked away, in a corner of my heart, will forever be such sweet gratitude for my dear friend and the spark that started it all.

Shortly after that revelation, the Law of Attraction stepped in and did its thing. That's when I met my two mentors, who would become special lifelong buddies. Celeste Rachell had been a doula and childbirth educator for many years when she entered my life. She was a true pioneer. I loved her from the moment I met her, for she embodied the kind of birth professional I wanted to be – just enough "crunchy" at her core, with a perfect mix of strength, affection, ingenuity, and business savvy. Every day since then, I pray I have made her proud. Ann Visser, accountant turned midwife, took me under her wing without hesitation when she was still teaching classes and going to births as a doula. She lovingly pushed me into the operating room (where people used to give birth whether or not they were having surgery) for my first doula stint. We called our alliance Partners In Birth and described ourselves as "professional labor assistants" at a time when no one knew what a doula was. She has been my enduring inspiration ever since.

Throughout the years I have learned from and leaned on an extensive, magnificent circle of birth sisters. I am extraordinarily lucky to be part of a special club of deep-feeling, mission-oriented souls who share a distinct calling. I will continue to marvel at how we could be left in a room for hours on end, and never run out of pregnancy and birth topics to discuss. The collective passion of these amazing women has energized my path.

To my students who have shared the most important, sensitive, personal, anxiety-provoking, joyful experience of their lives with me, I am humbled, honored, and indebted. They have welcomed me into the creation of their birth stories. They trusted me to guide them as those incredible, transformational stories unfolded. Their confidence in me fostered the courage I needed to write this book.

APPRECIATION

I began the composition of *The Ultimate Birth Experience* by gathering the reflections of many people who were willing to be surveyed and interviewed. I am grateful for their contributions of effort and enthusiasm. Without hesitation, many gave their time and their hearts to divulge their stories with the intention of offering lessons to my eventual readers. In particular, I thank the wonderful Jessica Dennehy, Scott Hartinger, Robyn and Jeff Lanci, Kaitlin McGreyes, DJ Meijer, Kara and Steven Szarek and Liana Watral. I must also give a special shout-out to Christina Kocis who not only meticulously scoured the manuscript for medical/technical/contextual accuracy, but graciously offered up real-life approaches to her superior midwifery care and agreed to write the foreword to this book without hesitation. And to my former student turned friend, Erin Meijer, my muse in many ways, who generously took the time to edit for content, advising me on inclusions by invoking the real and genuine voices of her peers - this book would not have come together the way it has without her input, and the exuberant, passionate support that she gave to this project and always bestows upon me.

Kimberly Turbin, who has told her story more times than I imagine she has cared to, graciously agreed to tell it yet again to me. All I had to do was make the request, and she was willing to answer every question I asked. I felt her trust in me and agonized over making sure that the message I connected to her story would both help others and further ensure that her traumatic experience did not occur in vain. I will say a simple thank-you, for I don't know that there are appropriate words of appreciation to convey to someone who bares their soul.

To have just one friend who loves and supports you, even when you are following a separate journey that they may not feel drawn to, is what good fortune is all about. I have many friends like that - friends who encourage my authenticity and champion all my endeavors. Friends who understood my need to isolate when this book was temporarily consuming my life. Friends who are like family. I am not only fortunate. I am blessed.

I worked on this book for two-and-a-half years before I was able to collect my voice, my intentions, and my focus. If not for Natasa and Stuart Denman, and everyone at *The Ultimate 48-Hour Author*, including Vivi, Julie and Lendy, I would still be in the weeds. I honestly don't know how anyone has ever written a book without their amazing guidance.

When I was a little girl, I used to have a fair share of anxiety around test-taking. My creative coping strategy was a simple reminder that no matter how poorly I might perform on a test, I would still grow up, get married and have babies. And so I did. I somehow knew that this would be the infrastructure of my accomplishments, my happiness and my legacy. What I could not have known was the extent to which I would be adored, and unconditionally supported by these 4 people who would comprise my nucleus. My children - Shane, Kendall, and Madison - are my reason for everything, and my husband, Scott, is my ally, my biggest fan, and my most cherished love. This book that I longed to write would never have been born without their endless encouragement and their unwavering belief in the realization of my dream.

REFERENCES

(1) Grant, Z. S., Wooding, S., & Grant, J. (2011). The answer is 17 years, what is the question: understanding time lags in translational research. *Journal of the Royal Society of Medicine*, 104(12) 510-520. https://www.ncbi.nlm. nih.gov/pmc/articles/PMC3241518/#:~:text=It%20is%20frequently%20 stated%20that,evidence%20to%20reach%20clinical%20practice.

(2) American Cancer Society. DES Exposure: Questions and Answers. Retrieved from https://www.cancer.org/cancer/cancer-causes/medical-treatments/ des-exposure.html

(3) United States Department of Health and Human Services, Centers for Disease Control and Prevention. DES History. Retrieved from https://www. cdc.gov/des/consumers/about/history.html#:~:text=The%20FDA%20 warning%20was%20based,birth%20(in%20the%20womb).

(4) Vargesson, N. (2015). Thalidomide-induced teratogenesis: History and mechanisms. *Birth Defects Res C Embryo Today*, 105(2) 140-156. https://www. ncbi.nlm.nih.gov/pmc/articles/PMC4737249/

(5) Mendes, E. 2014, January 9. The Study That Helped Spur the U.S. Stop-Smoking Movement. *American Cancer Society.* https://www.cancer.org/ latest-news/the-study-that-helped-spur-the-us-stop-smoking-movement. html

(6) Benson, C. B., & Doubilet, P. M. (2014). The History of Imaging in Obstetrics. *The Radiological Society of North America*. Retrieved from https://pubs. rsna.org/doi/full/10.1148/radiol.14140238

(7) Cunningham FG, Bangdiwala S, Brown SS, Dean TM, Frederiksen M, Rowland Hogue CJ, King T, Spencer Lukacz E, McCullough LB, Nicholson W, Petit N, Probstfield JL, Viguera AC, Wong CA, Zimmet SC. National Institutes of Health Consensus Development Conference Statement: Vaginal Birth After Cesarean: New Insights. March 8—10, 2010. Obstetrics & Gynecology. 2010; 115(6):1279–1295.

(8) Association of Ontario Midwives. Clinical Practice Guideline 14: Vaginal Birth after Previous Low-Segment Caesarean Section (September 2011). Retrieved from https://www.ontariomidwives.ca/vbac

(9) Kamel, J. 2020, February 24. New study reveals surprising truths behind the top three VBAC calculators. *VBAC Facts*. Retrieved from https://vbacfacts. com/2020/02/24/new-research-vbac-calculators/

(10) Obstetric Care Consensus. Safe Prevention of the Primary Cesarean Delivery (March 2014). Retrieved from https://www.acog.org/ clinical/clinical-guidance/obstetric-care-consensus/articles/2014/03/ safe-prevention-of-the-primary-cesarean-delivery

BONUS

Take the Birth IQ Quiz!

momsontop.com/birth-iq-quiz

As referenced in Chapter 2, the Birth IQ Quiz can be a tool, a roadmap, an initial passage toward expanding your knowledge about birth facts and actionable steps that could easily change the course of your labor.

Find out what you know and what you may not know about:

o The signposts of impending labor
o The most important role of the support coach
o What to do if labor stalls because your baby is not descending and how to apply the answers as you work toward achieving your ultimate birth experience!

Download *The Ultimate Guide for Empowered Moms*

momsontop.com/guide-for-empowered-moms

The perfect time to begin preparing for motherhood is when you're preparing for birth.

The Ultimate Guide for Empowered Moms will lay the groundwork for a healthy, confident, self-assured mindset as you transition into motherhood, or continue on your path.

Learn how to sharpen your mind, strengthen your body, and empower your spirit in each of the areas of the Moms On Top Wellness Wheel, such as:

- o Fitness
- o Nutrition
- o Parenting
- o Relationships
- o Personal development

and more!

Don't miss this chance to point your life as a mom in the direction of empowerment!

GAIL JANICOLA

is the author of The Ultimate Birth Experience and the founder of Moms On Top, a resource for unbiased, evidence-based education and coaching, serving moms from "pre-nest to empty nest". She has been speaking on the subject of pregnancy, childbirth, and wellness for over 25 years.

To further her natural coaching skills, Gail formally trained with the Functional Medicine Coaching Academy and went on to become a National Board Certified Health and Wellness Coach.

Gail has been interviewed extensively in media sources on subjects such as Normalizing Birth: Making Birth Your Own in Today's Medical System, and What I Wish I Knew Sooner – A Must Watch For Moms-to-Be.

An in-demand and captivating speaker, Gail teaches and coaches what she has lived. Her no-nonsense honesty allows her to connect with her audience from the heart, engaging them with her genuine, nurturing, non-judgmental style. As one colleague put it, "Gail has a warm, loving, endless energy to her that wraps you up the moment you are in her presence."

How to take control of your birth experience and proactively choose the options that are best for you and your baby:

o Assembling your birth team

o Advocating, and communicating with medical care providers

o Choosing wisely from the "Natural Bag" and the "Medical Bag"

From Overwhelmed to Overjoyed – A mother's path to empowerment and lifelong happiness:

o 3 P's: Perspective, Priority, Purpose

o The physical/mental health connection: How mental health influences physical health and physical health influences mental health

o Stop resenting your partner and get the support you need

Courageously Parenting Children, Teens and Young Adults:

o Moving from rescuing and fixing to accepting and validating

o Not losing yourself in the difficult process of parenting

o Managing the extreme emotions and frequent fallout when a child struggles

To inquire about engaging Gail to speak at your next event, please contact
info@momsontop.com or
516.848.9028
for prices and availabilities.

203

ABOUT THE AUTHOR

Gail Janicola became a Certified Childbirth Educator and a Certified Doula in 1995, shortly after the births of her first two children. She is also a National Board Certified Health and Wellness Coach, the Doula trainer for Long Island Doula Association, and the founder of Moms On Top, a resource for unbiased, evidence-based education, coaching, and support, serving moms throughout the parenting life cycle, from "pre-nest to empty nest".

Gail has been cited in several media sources such as Aaptiv, Baby Gaga, and Mommee Friends, and interviewed for various birth, health, and lifestyle platforms, including The Fearless Family Health podcast and Mom Life TV. She currently teaches, coaches and speaks nationwide.

Gail lives on Long Island (New York) with her devoted, supportive husband and their fur baby, Baci. She has three grown children who are the light of her life.

Additional Thoughts and Actions

_____

_____

_____

_____

_____

_____

_____

_____

_____

_____

_____

_____

_____

_____

Additional Thoughts and Actions

_____

_____

_____

_____

_____

_____

_____

_____

_____

_____

_____

_____

_____

Additional Thoughts and Actions

CPSIA information can be obtained
at www.ICGtesting.com
Printed in the USA
FSHW010956140421
80454FS